# A Healer In Every Home

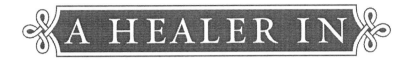

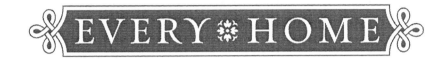

# QuickStart Edition

Begabati Lennihan RN, CCH

GreenHealing

**GreenHealing Productions**
777 Concord Ave. Suite 301
Cambridge, Mass. 02138
www.greenhealing.org

ISBN 978-0-9834431-0-0

Back cover photo: Lydia Knutson, DC
Cover design: Ron Frank

**Disclaimer:** It is advisable to seek the guidance of a physician before implementing the approach to health suggested in this book. It is essential that any reader who has any reason to suspect that he or she suffers from illness check with his or her doctor before attempting to treat it with this method. Neither this nor any other book should be used as a substitute for professional medical care or treatment.

**Acknowledgements:** In this field even more so than others, a book like this is based on layer upon layer of knowledge gleaned from generations of practitioners, teachers and writers who have come before.
My most direct inspiration for this book is from Luc De Schepper, Catherine Coulter, Dana Ullman and Miranda Castro. I studied their teachings many years ago and have refrained from consulting their works again while writing this book, in order to avoid unconsciously copying them.

This book is the fruit of my own experience; if I have unwittingly imitated my teachers, it is because the truth of their teaching was borne out in my practice.

I would also like to thank the thousands of customers in my health food store, the hundreds of clients in my practice and students in my schools, and especially the faculty members of Teleosis School of Homeopathy – Peris Gumz, RN,CCH; Loretta Butehorn, PhD, CCH; Tanya Renner, CCH; and Kim Kalina, CCH, RSHom(NA), for all that I learned from them about how to teach.

## Dedication

To my parents –
my father the doctor and my mother the teacher,
nature lovers both,
who gave me a wildflower garden when I was little
and with it a love for the healing powers of plants


and to Sri Chinmoy, my spiritual teacher,
who loved homeopathy,
learned to use it as a youth in India,
and inspired me to become a homeopath.

Hi there! This is your quick-start guide to treating yourself, your family and even your beloved pets with safe, effective natural remedies.

Along the way, we'll introduce you to the top remedies you'll want to have on hand in your home medicine chest.

This book is based on my years of running a health food store – a small store where I talked to thousands of customers about what they were buying and why, about what worked, and how they could tell that it worked.

A couple of things surprised me.
One was that people could not actually feel vitamins and other supplements working.

Now don't get me wrong – I think that vitamins and supplements are really important. If people ask, "Why can't I just get what I need from food?" I would give them the same answer now that I used to give back then:

Definitely you can get all the nutrients you need from food! You just have to be willing to grow all your food in your own back yard, fertilize it with organic compost, and eat it right after it is picked – because the vitamin content goes downhill quickly when fruits and vegetables are picked.

Plus you have to avoid all the things that drain nutrients from your system – everything from sugar and alcohol to fluorescent lights to stress. And avoid all the sources of toxins in our world, since vitamins and other supplements help protect against toxins – so you have to avoid polluted air and water and many things made out of plastic.

If you can't commit to that lifestyle – you do need vitamins!

But here's the other thing I found fascinating.

There was one type of remedy I sold in my store that when my customers took it – often they would open the tube and take it right at the checkout counter – they would often say, "WOW! Could it work that fast?"

What was doubly amazing was that hardly anyone knew about these remedies. Here I was within a mile of Harvard University, with probably the most highly educated clientele of any health food store in the country, customers who were avid readers about anything related to natural healing – and just a few of them seemed to know about these remedies that worked so quickly and dramatically.

When I turned 40, I decided to sell the store and study professionally the modality that worked the most dramatically for my customers – it's called homeopathy, "home – ee – OP – uh – thee".

You can definitely say this – it starts with the word "home"!

So in this book I'll be sharing the top tips that I gleaned in my store and in my professional practice – primarily using remedies from homeopathy (the little sugar pellets, different from herbs) because they're so safe, so effective, and it's hard to find this kind of information anywhere else.

I still believe in the value of vitamins, minerals and herbs – they provide the body with the raw materials it needs, while homeopathic remedies restore the body's blueprint.

But information about herbs and supplements is so plentiful and easily available that I decided to focus here on homeopathy plus my favorite things from the health food store – things you might not know about otherwise.

That way you'll get the "biggest bang from this book."

Okay, let's get started! My name is Begabati – I've taught hundreds of people to use these remedies and handed out thousands of remedies myself – now I'm looking forward to being of service to you.

More about me, my unusual name and my passion for natural healing at www.greenhealing.org – there's a short 3-minute video on the home page where I introduce myself.

**Helpful links:** we have lots of useful links in this book. Send us an email at books@greenhealing.org and we'll email you the links so you can access them easily.

We'll also let you know about our new books as they become available – like the guide for natural pet care, and the Professional Version of this book, designed to send to your doctor if she or he says these natural remedies are "unproven." It will be full of references to scientific studies that may help make doctors more open minded to natural healing.

## How to use this book

Each section contains

o   a **condition** to be treated

o   a top **remedy** to get acquainted with

o   one or more **scenarios** of what might happen as you use the remedies

o   **supplemental things** you can get at the health food store

o   and other **quick tips**.

For your convenience each type of item is grouped together on its own page in the Table of Contents.

# Contents

Introduction: Let's Get Started ........................... 1

"Help, Mom!" First Aid Remedies ...................... 5

Bumps, Bruises and Sports Injuries ..................... 14

Cuts, Scrapes and Surgery .................................. 21

"Mommy, I'm Bleeding!" .................................. 28

"Ouch, My Nerve Endings!" ............................... 32

Emotional First Aid ........................................... 36

Drippy with a Cold ........................................... 45

Droopy with a Flu ............................................. 57

Sick to Your Stomach? ....................................... 67

Stings and Hives ............................................... 77

Sprains, Strains and Creaky Joints ....................... 82

Teething .......................................................... 89

Resource Section .............................................. 97
*continued on next page*

## Resource Section

Cell Salts (Tissue Salts) ............................................. 98

Safety Guidelines ..................................................... 85

Partner With Your Doctor ........................................ 89

Find a Doctor to Partner With ............................... 91

Find a Professional Homeopath .............................. 93

How the Remedies Work ........................................ 95

What to Say to a Skeptic ......................................... 97

Diving Deeper – Reference Materials ...................... 99

Books to Enjoy Reading ........................................ 101

Books on Specific Topics ....................................... 103

Websites to Explore .............................................. 104

Support Your Body's Healing Energy ................... 105

Index ..................................................................... 110

## "Make Friends with the Remedies" Overview

Here is where you can find in-depth information about these remedies – probably the **first remedies** to stock in your home medicine chest, both because they are **used the most,** and also because they are apt to be used **in emergency situations** – in other words, when you don't have time to go out and buy them.

Aconite ............................................................. 9

Arnica ............................................................. 15

Calendula ...................................................... 21

Phosphorus ................................................... 29

Hypericum ..................................................... 33

Ignatia ........................................................... 40

Arsenicum ..................................................... 52

Gelsemium .................................................... 62

Nux vomica .................................................... 70

Apis ................................................................ 78

Rhus tox ........................................................ 83

Bryonia .......................................................... 84

Pulsatilla ........................................................ 91

## "Health Food Store Helpers" Overview

These are just a few favorite supplemental products from the health food store. There are so many wonderful things in your health food store that I can't begin to cover them all – plus the information about most of them is easily available. In a world of TMI (too much information), I just picked out a few favorites, including a few things that may not have made it to your local store yet – please tell your store staff about them!

First Aid.............................................................. 7

Bumps, Bruises, and Sports Injuries................... 14

Frazzled Nerves ............................................... 34

Emotional First Aid .......................................... 43

Colds and the Immune System ......................... 51

Flu.................................................................... 59

Stings and Hives.............................................. 80

Joint Pain ....................................................... 85

Teething.......................................................... 95

## "Now What?" Overview

These are the different scenarios of what might happen after you give a remedy – or while you are still trying to figure out how to give the first dose! I've found it's easier to understand these "followup scenarios" if they're given in context – so I've sprinkled them throughout the book.

At some point you might want to come back and study them all at one fell swoop, so they are listed here for your convenience.

Actually that would be a good idea, because it's hard to focus on this kind of thing "in the heat of the moment."

Can I take more than one remedy at a time?.................. 8

My pre-surgery instructions say Nothing By Mouth......... 26

How do I give the remedies after surgery? ..................... 27

The symptoms stopped. Now what do I do? .................. 31

My friend doesn't want to numb her grief with drugs.... 41

I'm no better but my symptoms have changed.............. 56

My child fell asleep after taking the remedy .................. 63

No change after three doses of the remedy................... 73

I'm no better but my symptoms have changed, part 2.... 87

My symptoms keep getting worse................................. 92

## Quick Tips Overview

Safe for Babies ...................................................... 17

Safety First .......................................................... 19

Remedies for Surgery and Tooth Extractions ........ 22

If It Has an Alcohol Base ....................................... 44

Making the Remedies Stronger ............................. 47

Hypersensitives ..................................................... 49

Giving the Remedies in Water .............................. 50

"Nip It in the Bud" ................................................ 60

Put Together a Travel Kit ....................................... 76

Splinters and Fungal Nails .................................... 80

Pulsatilla for Pets .................................................. 92

# Let's Get Started

Before we start, here are the basic principles on which this book is founded. I bet you'll like them!

1. **Empowerment:** putting the power in your hands to heal yourself and your family – of course when appropriate.

2. **Be the expert in your own body.** You *are* the expert! Have you ever tried to tell a doctor that you were in pain or something was wrong, and your doctor said it was all in your head? You *know* when something is wrong with your body, and you *know* when you feel something is working. This book asks you to notice your body, in sickness and in health, and it honors your own sense of your body.

3. **Partner with your doctor** – and find a doctor to partner with, who respects your interest in natural healing. More about this on pages 104–107, but in the meantime – remember your doctor is really busy and doesn't have as much time as you do, to study natural healing. The great majority of doctors are dedicated and compassionate healers who are understandably skeptical about what they don't know. Help them out by sharing your success stories.

4. **Take responsibility for your health.** Too many people plop themselves in the doctor's office after eating a junk food diet and not exercising and say, "Fix me." This is too much to expect! You need to take responsibility for yourself.

5. **First do no harm.** This is actually the first line in the oath of healing that doctors take! The best medicine to start with is the one likely to do the most good with the least risk of harm – which is exactly what the remedies in this book are all about – a 200 year track record of safety, even in infants.

## Buying the remedies – it's easy and inexpensive

New to this? just dipping your toe in the water?
You can buy these remedies as the need comes up,
from any health food store, some drug stores, and online.
They typically cost about $7 for enough to last a long time.

We recommend getting them from Homeopathic Educational
Services, **www.homeopathic.com**, because the site also
has so much useful information.

Ready to roll up your sleeves and really dig in?
Better yet, buy a kit of remedies:

- o  you'll save hundreds of dollars in the long run

- o  you'll have the remedies on hand in the middle
     of the night when you need them

- o  the pellets are tiny and dissolve easily in water

- o  you get 1500 pellets in each tube, very economical

- o  the kit is so compact, it's easy to travel with.

We recommend the First Aid Emergency Kit of 50 remedies
from Natural Health Supply, **www.a2zhomeopathy.com.**
Get them in the 30c potency (strength) – the most common
strength to use for home care – and in the small (half dram)
size.

**Questions?** email us at books@greenhealing.org.
Can't promise to answer them all, but we may refer to them
in an upcoming blog, or use them to improve this book next
time around.

Keep **checking the blog** at www.greenhealing.org for answers to yours and other folks' questions.

Also check out our YouTube channel!

**GreenHealingTV on YouTube.**
In the videos we demonstrate things that are hard to describe in a book – infant massage, yoga for pregnancy, a daily energy routine, and much more.

**Feedback? success stories?**
email us at <u>books@greenhealing.org</u>.
If we use your material in the next edition, we'll send you a free copy with our thanks.

**Full disclosure:**
We recommend lots of products in this book, and we have NO financial interest in any of them, except the *Healer In Every Home* books, and the *Mastering Natural Remedies* video series which we produced with leading homeopath Miranda Castro, available on our site, <u>www.greenhealing.org.</u>

# "Help, Mom!" First Aid Remedies

Your five year old insists on "helping" in the kitchen, grabs a knife when you're distracted for a moment, thinks she's cut herself and is screaming bloody murder – except there's no blood, she's just scared.

You've just had a fender bender – or a near miss and your heart is racing a mile a minute because it was such a close call!

Your elderly mother calls – she's terrified because she's having heart palpitations.

**What do you do RIGHT AWAY?**

Call 911, of course, if the situation warrants it –

but what do you do for your five year old?

or if you didn't actually have a car accident, just a close call that left you terrified?

Answer – give **ACONITE!**
the first remedy to get for your home medicine chest.

If you do need to call 911, you can give Aconite while waiting for the ambulance.

**ACONITE** is probably the most important of these natural remedies to have on hand, just in case – because when you need it, there won't be time to order it online or try to find it in a health food store.

Aconite is for an **emergency** that just happened

o    or for **a close call**

o    or for a situation when the person feels like they **almost died or could die**

o    when they are in a **total panic** and their **heart is racing**.


It will help calm them down so they can focus their body's healing energies on the situation at hand.

Or if you're the one that needs it – it helps you pull yourself together and **think clearly in an emergency**.

It's likely to **calm a racing heart in a panic situation** – and that helps break the vicious cycle of fear which makes your heart race, which makes you even more afraid.

Of course, if you are having an actual heart attack, it won't fix that, which is why you need to use common sense and call 911 when needed.

So if you'd like to start slowly and get these remedies one at a time – we suggest starting with Aconite.

(And if you have family members far away who are open to using natural remedies – get some Aconite for them too. Maybe even get an extra to keep in your glove compartment, since cars are a typical place where you might need it.)

# Health Food Store Helpers for First Aid

**RESCUE REMEDY** is another remedy to have on hand for situations like this.

It's a blend of five Flower Essences – remedies based on flower power!
Who could imagine that a simple solution distilled from flowers could be so powerful?

But if you get some at the health food store and keep it on hand, you'll see for yourself how quickly it can work in emergency situations.

Rescue Remedy is worth a try for all kinds of **traumas,** whether **physical injury** or **emotional shock** – anything that "just happened" and leaves the person trembling or upset.

It can even heal physical wounds.

At the very least Aconite and Rescue Remedy can buy you some time while you get appropriate medical help – and calm a screaming child in the meantime.

You'll need to get Rescue Remedy in a health food store – it doesn't come in a remedy kit.

# Now what?

"I took the Aconite and I'm much calmer – but I'm really hurt! Now what should I take? And can I take two remedies at the same time?"

We're getting to that – remedies for cuts, bruises, and so forth – in later chapters.

Use common sense and our Safety Guidelines (see page 99) to decide whether it's something you can treat at home or if it needs medical help.

Normally you take just one remedy at a time, because it's giving your body information and you don't want to confuse it. Just one remedy on a given day is a good rule of thumb.

In an emergency you might actually need more than one remedy at a time. Start with the one that's most urgent.

You can give a dose of **Sulphur** before changing remedies. Sulphur is like clearing the palate or resetting the dials. It gets the body ready for the next remedy.

Definitely don't put two remedies in the mouth at the same time, unless you're using a combination remedy from the health food store. These remedies are so low potency that they seem to work fine together.

It's like this: giving a remedy is like dropping a pebble into a pond, as my friend Miranda Castro would say. A good remedy spreads its ripples (its effects) to the whole pond. Another pebble would create different ripples and an interference pattern.

A low-potency combination is like several small pebbles with little ripples that don't touch each other. Rescue Remedy is also fine to take with other remedies, because it's so mild

# Make Friends with ACONITE

We'll be encouraging you to learn about the remedies
one at a time – with **simple key words** or phrases for each
one to help you get a handle on all the many conditions
that each one can be used for.

That's one of the great things about this system –
each remedy can be used for so many different things!

and by the way, only of these many uses can fit on a
remedy label. That's why the remedy you use for your
sore throat might say "hot flashes"!

So you get a lot of mileage out of each little tube you buy,
and out of each remedy you get to know.

Here are your **key words for Aconite** –
it can be used when several of these themes are present:

o  **sudden** – for conditions that come on all of a sudden

o  **fright** – used when the person is "scared to death" or
   "almost died" or feels like "I'm afraid I'll die from this!"

o  **restless** and **anxious**

o  **heart** – often there are heart palpitations

o  **cold wind** – it can also be used for infectious things that
   come on after a cold wind – for example, kids playing
   outside in winter, they start to sweat under their heavy
   coats, then a wind comes up, they get chilled and get
   sick

o  **middle of the night** – when someone wakes up sick in
   the middle of the night, often after being chilled during
   the day

Put these together and you get conditions like these:

- o bladder infections
- o colds
- o conjunctivitis
- o croup
- o ear infections
- o fever
- o flu
- o laryngitis
- o measles
- o sore throat

when one or more of these conditions is present: sudden onset; after a fright; with fearfulness and restlessness; the person wakes up with it

and most often used at the **first stage** of the illness – that's why you need to have it on hand!

**Special uses:** when your eye hurts because it had a foreign object in it, Aconite will help.

By the way – do you know this trick for getting something out of your eye?
Pull your upper lid away from the eye, pull it up towards the top of your eye, then touch your eye with it and sweep it down touching your eye – a lot of times this will get that pesky little thing out.

**So remember, for Aconite –**

- o sudden
- o fright /fearful and restless
- o heart
- o cold wind
- o middle of the night

that's all you need to remember!

# Bumps, Bruises and Sports Injuries

o   Your two-year-old just toppled off her high chair.

o   Your seven-year-old just fell off his skateboard.

o   Your thirteen-year-old pulled a muscle playing soccer

o   Your seventeen-year-old feels "beat up" after a
    football game.

o   Your best friend just got a nose job and now she can't go
    out of the house because her face is all black and blue.

Use **ARNICA** for all these situations and you may feel like a
miracle worker.

Lots of people have told us that they had no bruising after
plastic surgery – just by using Arnica! in fact, many plastic
surgeons themselves are now using Arnica because they get
better results.

What do all these conditions have in common?

o   a **blow or trauma** – can be from falling,
    from a sports injury, from surgery

o   often you can see a **bruise** forming

o   the person often reports **feeling sore, beaten up**, or
    **bruised**

o   there may be **swelling** from fluid leaking from broken
    blood vessels

11

## What to do?

First consider whether you need emergency medical help
[see Safety First, page 19, and Safety Guidelines, page 99].

Then get your Arnica, from your kit or medicine cabinet or
local health food store.

## How to give the remedies
Typically you would give **two pellets every four hours**
as long as the symptoms are INTENSE (injury just happened,
really hurts) then **twice a day** when the person is on the
mend.

STOP giving the remedy as soon as they are better.

In an emergency, give as often as **every 15 minutes**.

## Story Time

I was helping a friend babysit for his four-year-old daughter while his wife was out for the evening. His little girl ran into the livingroom, skidded on the rug, tripped over the dog, and banged her forehead on the corner of the piano bench. Ouch!

Her forehead started to swell visibly and she soon had a goose-egg the size of half a baseball.

We gave her Arnica and the goose-egg disappeared as quickly as it had appeared!

A pharmacist friend decided to do an experiment when she got a large bruise. She rubbed Arnica cream on half of it, which went away immediately, leaving the other untreated half to turn shades of green and purple for a week.

You might want to try this too. Do your own science experiment on yourself!

# Health Food Store Helpers for Bruises

Arnica can also be applied externally –
in fact a great way to do that is by using **Traumeel** ointment,
a wonderful combination of Arnica and other remedies that
are good for traumas and injuries.

If someone bruises easily, it could mean that the walls of
their blood vessels are too fragile.

They may need to **strengthen the walls of their
blood vessels,** and they can safely try doing that with:

o **Calc fluor 6x,** a tissue salt (see p. 98) for
  strengthening elastic tissues like blood vessel walls –
  this also helps people who sprain their ankles easily,
  because it strengthens connective tissue in general.
  Get the 6x strength and dissolve two tablets in your
  mouth twice a day. They dissolve easily and taste
  sweet.

o **Rutin**, part of the vitamin C complex

o or **eat foods high in rutin** like
  – the white on the inside of an orange peel;
  – black tea;
  – and buckwheat or kasha
    (this is a fabulous source of plant-based protein and
    would be a great addition to your meals anyway).

# Make friends with ARNICA

This is one of those remedies that belongs in every medic.. ie cabinet – and in every gym bag, along with its friend **Traumeel** the topical ointment.

If you can remember these three key symptoms, you'll know how to use it:

o **bruised**

o **soft tissue trauma**

o **"I'm fine! Leave me alone"**

It's perfect for those times when people have been injured and the endorphins (natural painkillers) come out and they **don't feel pain** – but you're looking at them and you know they're hurt!

It also works for a variety of conditions where there hasn't been an actual blow –
but the person feels bruised, sore or beaten up –
sometimes this happens with **the flu**,
and sometimes with **jet lag**.

So here's a list of what it's useful for – you don't have to remember the list, just remember the three keys to Arnica:

o after childbirth for mother and baby
   especially if the baby has a bruise on its head

o black eyes

o bruises

o concussion – of course with appropriate medical help

o dental extractions – see p. 22

o flu

o jet lag

o nosebleeds especially after a blow to the nose

o sore muscles

o sports injuries – pulled muscles

o surgery – see p. 22

## Story Time

Soccer superstar David Beckham uses Arnica – along with many of the top sports teams and athletes in Europe. American athletes are starting to catch on as well. Read about them and all the top celebrities using homeopathy in the fascinating book *The Homeopathic Revolution* by Dana Ullman.

# Quick Tip: Safe for Babies!

These remedies have been used safely for 200 years now for millions of people – including babies.

The FDA has approved them for babies and small children! Just be careful that your baby doesn't choke on a remedy pellet.

Here's how to avoid that:

o   If you get the kit from Natural Health Supply (see p. 2), the pellets are tiny, like a grain of sand, and you can safely tuck one inside your baby's mouth.

o   If you get a "blue tube" from the health food store, the pellets are bigger, the size of a pea, so you'll need to crush them into a powder and put a bit into your baby's mouth, or dissolve in a little water

o   You can also dab this water onto your baby's lips or even onto the temples –
    the remedy will absorb through the delicate skin –
    and you may feel more comfortable applying the remedy externally instead of putting something into your baby's mouth, especially if you're new to these remedies (and/or new to being a parent!)

You'll feel more comfortable with these remedies as you become more experienced and discover how safe they are.

# BRF: Best Remedy Friends, Arnica and Bellis

Some remedies have a "best friend" –
a remedy that acts as a "backup" if the first remedy doesn't
work.

Arnica has a great "best friend" called **Bellis**.
If Arnica doesn't work when you think it should,
try Bellis.

Also, there are a few situations where
**Bellis works even better than Arnica:**

o   for soft tissue trauma to the **chest, breast, abdomen**.

o   Think **mammograms**!
    You know painful they are?
    Try a dose of Bellis before and after.

o   Or think of a high-school girl athlete who gets a
    fast ball right to the breast – ouch!

o   Also, for the bruised sore feeling **after childbirth**,
    or **after abdominal surgery,**
    Arnica will work great!
    and Bellis may work even better.

# Quick Tip: Safety First!

Sometimes people get so passionate about natural healing, they avoid doctors and hospitals at all costs.

But we need doctors and hospitals! There are some things that just can't be treated at home.

Please use common sense and don't go overboard.

In an emergency situation where you would have called 911, gone to the emergency room, or called your doctor before you learned about natural healing – **still do that!**

One of the most important situations is when someone has hit their head and is having

o  loss of consciousness and/or seizures (convulsions)

o  prolonged dizziness and/or vomiting

o  headache and/or confusion.

Please see a more complete list of safety guidelines on page 99.

BUMPS, BRUISES, SPORTS INJURIES o ARNICA

## Story Time

A nurse who was studying homeopathy with me called me for a remedy suggestion, saying, "I know my little boy has appendicitis but I don't want to take him to the hospital because I'm afraid they will give him antibiotics and that will mess up his system."

I said, "Take him to the hospital! The antibiotics could save his life! We can do something about the antibiotics later!"

I refrained from saying, "Are you crazy?"

Please don't be too fanatical about natural remedies!

# Cuts, Scrapes and Surgery

Anytime the skin is broken or cut, **Calendula** is your best friend. It does several important things:

o   **knits together** the two sides of a cut

o   helps **prevent infection**

o   **reduces pain**

o   **prevents scarring**

How to give Calendula:
If you have a kit, you have it in pellet form.
It will work well taken internally – it works throughout the whole body at the same time.

**In water:**
You can also dissolve a few pellets in a half-cup of water and apply it externally.
You can pour it over the wound and/or soak the bandage in Calendula water.
So the pellets give you a lot of flexibility for both internal and external use – and you'll probably get quicker results if you use it both ways.

If you don't have a kit, though, you probably won't find the pellets in a health food store. You can easily find

**Calendula cream, Calendula lotion, Calendula spray**

– the spray is especially good for applying to a very tender area, say a burn, where you don't want to touch it to smear something on.

# Quick Tip: Remedies for Surgery and Tooth Extractions

Maybe the most dramatic use for your new remedy friends is before and after surgery or a tooth extraction.

You can take a dose of **Arnica** and a dose of **Calendula** preventively right beforehand,
and additional doses as needed afterwards.

One more remedy for pre-and post-surgery: **PHOSPHORUS**.

Used preventively, it helps protect against the effects of anesthesia – for anyone who has a past history of not coming out of anesthesia easily.

Are you the type of person who needs to be "slapped to wake up" from anesthesia?

For you, it's especially important to take a dose of Phosphorus ahead of time.

Phosphorus also helps control bleeding – especially useful after a tooth extraction.

See the next chapter, "Mommy, I'm Bleeding!" for more about Phosphorus.

## Story Time

When I first studied homeopathy, there was a dentist in the class who started giving his patients Calendula before he performed oral surgery. He said he could see the incision healing (or as he put it, "granulation tissue forming") right before his eyes!

## Story Time

I've had some dramatic results with the pre- and post-surgery protocol:

One of my students used it for her mother, who was in her 80s and was in the hospital for bowel resection surgery – in other words, her abdomen would be cut open and part of her bowel removed, then the parts stitched together – so it involved lots of cutting – a very painful kind of surgery!

Now I remember from my nursing school days, part of our job was to try to get patients up out of bed after surgery and walking a few steps, on a schedule prescribed by the doctor …

… and I remember how hard it was to do that, especially with elderly people.

It would be so painful for them to move, they just wanted to lie there and save their energy.

Do you know, this elderly lady, the day after her surgery (according to her daughter) shocked her nurses by climbing over the bedrails and walking to the bathroom by herself!

One of my clients told me a similar story. Her mother, sadly, needed a double mastectomy; my client asked me for the surgery remedies for her mom.

After an operation like this, patients typically get pain medication on a schedule, plus they can dispense extra pain medication when they need it.

The nurses were amazed that even after having both breasts removed (can you imagine how painful that would be?) this woman did not use any of her additional pain medication.

I've heard many similar stories, from my clients and students, of using the surgery remedies and having the surgeon afterwards comment afterwards that it was her or his "best work" because the incision healed so beautifully with minimal pain and scarring.

Unfortunately, none of the patients told the surgeon that they had used homeopathic remedies – they let the surgeon take the credit!

I hope that you will share with your doctor the results you get from using these remedies.

Doctors need to hear from you – it will help create the "partnership" with doctors that we talk about on page 104.

The more people tell their doctors about their successes with natural healing, the more doctors will feel comfortable and familiar with the concept.

If you are afraid to tell your doctor because you are afraid of being criticized, maybe it's time to find a doctor who will listen to you respectfully (see Find Another Doctor, on page 106).

We need to create a change in the health care system in this country from the ground up – starting with people like you and me – a change based on safe, effective, inexpensive natural remedies used FIRST before high-tech, high-cost, potentially dangerous medical interventions.

Doctors are almost always people of great sincerity, compassion and integrity, and they have dedicated their lives to your healing – they want this change too but they don't know about this solution yet – they need to hear about it from you!

# Now what?

"I want to give the pre-surgery remedies but my instructions say Nothing By Mouth."

What they really mean is – they don't want people to swallow something before the operation which they might vomit up and then breathe into their lungs – big trouble!

The remedies dissolve in the mouth
**so you won't be swallowing anything.**

If you want to be follow your pre-surgery instructions literally, though, you can dissolve each remedy in a little water and dab it onto your lips, temples, inside of your wrists – your body's healing energy will still "get the message."

Because it's hard to give remedies in the hospital, it's best to take them before you leave for the hospital.

It might help to tell the hospital staff that these remedies are safe and FDA-regulated just like conventional medications – but honestly, it probably won't get you anywhere.

Some day, conventional doctors and hospitals will come to know what a wonderful, helpful and safe support these remedies are – and perhaps someday the remedies will be part of the before-and-after surgery protocol in every hospital.

In the meantime, we need to respect their restrictions, which are based on a concern for your safety and the need to protect people against unfamiliar substances.

## Now what?

"How do I give the remedies after the surgery?"

You'll most likely need to wait until the patient comes home because the staff will not allow you to give anything they are not familiar with.

(One way to get around this – dissolve the remedies in a small bottle of water and label it 'holy water'. Is it really holy water? Yes, if you believe it is. It is healing water, and healing is a sacred act. Nurses are trained to respect your religious beliefs and will treat your 'holy water' with respect.)

Give **Arnica** as long as there is bruising, soreness and swelling – maybe a few days.

Give **Calendula** (and soak the gauze with it) until the surgical incision is completely healed.

If you want to be sure to prevent scarring, use Miranda Castro's **Scar Cream** – not in shops yet but available online from www.mirandacastro.com.

Miranda tells me that her local plastic surgeon buys the cream from her 50 bottles at a time because he gets such good results with it!

By the way, before you go in for surgery please get *Prepare for Surgery, Heal Faster* by my old friend Peggy Huddleston. Peggy was a customer in my health food store while she was writing the book! The book and CD provide relaxation exercises that will help you be less anxious beforehand and also have less pain and recover more quickly afterwards.

# "Mommy, I'm Bleeding!"

o  a nosebleed that just won't stop

o  bleeding from a tooth extraction

o  a cut that just keeps on bleeding

o  profuse menstrual bleeding, if it's bright red

Any of these situations can benefit from **PHOSPHORUS** especially if it's bright red blood.

Some people bleed more easily than others, and have a harder time getting the bleeding to stop –

these people are often likely to need Phosphorus to control the bleeding.

Use common sense – is the bleeding potentially dangerous?

If so, use Phosphorus while on the way to conventional medical care.

# Make Friends With PHOSPHORUS

Phosphorus is a great remedy to have on hand.
Its uses are easy to remember – you just have to remember
three things about Phosphorus:

- o **bright red blood**
- o **dry cough, hoarseness, laryngitis**
- o **electrical shocks**

**Electrical shocks** might include

- o a shock from faulty wiring
- o touching an electrified fence
- o being hit by lightning.

Of course get appropriate medical help!

**Bright red bleeding,** just to review, can include
a wide variety of situations:

- o bleeding gums or bleeding after tooth extraction
- o bleeding hemorrhoids
- o cuts that just won't stop bleeding, or after surgery
- o coughing or vomiting blood
- o nosebleed
- o heavy menstrual bleeding
- o postpartum hemorrhage

Phosphorus might stop the bleeding or help control it while
you get appropriate medical help.

Phosphorus is also a great remedy for **dry coughs** – but coughs are tricky because there are so many good remedies for coughs.

If you have a dry cough, especially if it gets worse when you talk or go out in cold air, you can try Phosphorus for it.

But if it doesn't work, please don't say,
"These remedies don't work."
Just know that you probably need a different remedy.

Coughs are tricky because there are so many good cough remedies, so it's hard to pick the right one.

Get some experience and confidence with the easy situations in this book, and then move on to a more advanced book – see pages 114–119.

# Now what?

"My child's nosebleed stopped. Now what do I do?"

Stop the remedy!

These remedies work differently from conventional medicine. Like when you take antibiotics, you are told to complete the course, even if you feel better.

We'll tell you the opposite – STOP as soon as you feel better. We're just trying to give enough doses to get the ball rolling – the ball of healing, that is.

If you take too much of the remedy, it can boomerang and actually intensify the symptoms it's meant to cure. This is called an "aggravation".

This is a harmless result and it's actually part of the healing process – it means that too much of the remedy gave your body too hard a shove in the right direction.

Your body couldn't handle the surplus of "remedy-energy", and created symptoms.

When you stop the remedy, the symptoms will go away and you'll feel even better than before the remedy.

This rarely happens, though, with an acute condition (a short-lived condition you can treat at home).

In my own practice with hundreds of clients, I can only remember a couple of times that this happened with acute conditions.

So not to worry. Just be aware.

# "Ouch, My Nerve Endings!"

A favorite story from my childhood – my mom still laughs, remembering me when I was barely old enough to talk, stubbing a toe and (apparently showing an early interest in anatomy and physiology) saying "Ouch, my nerve endings!"

When you injure yourself in a nerve-rich area like a fingertip, toe, or lip, use **HYPERICUM** – the remedy for nerve injuries.

Another nerve-rich area is the base of the spine – so it can relieve the pain when someone slips and falls right on their "tush."

Remember to go to your chiropractor if it was a serious fall!

Another injury to a nerve-rich area: a tear or an episiotomy (a planned incision to allow for more stretching) during childbirth. Ouch, what a painful area! Hypericum will help.

Hypericum is also great for shooting pains which are likely to be along the path of a nerve – for example, sometimes people describe pain going from a tooth along a path like a thin line or a thin thread – they may get great relief from Hypericum.

It might even work for sciatica, which is pain along the sciatic nerve – especially if the person feels the pain shooting along the nerve (which goes down the leg)

So it's worth a try, but there are lots of other remedies for sciatica, so if Hypericum doesn't work, please seek help from a professional homeopath (see page 108).

# Make friends with HYPERICUM

This is an easy one! Two concepts –

– **crushed nerves**

– **nerve pain** (like pins and needles, or shooting along the path of a nerve

and that's all you need to know about Hypericum!


Examples:

- o   when you hit your finger with a hammer
- o   when you hit your lip
- o   a piercing on the lip, tongue or other tender area
- o   a tear or incision in the vaginal area during chldbirth
- o   puncture wounds
- o   injuries to the tailbone
- o   pain in the root of a tooth especially if it feels like a thin thread of pain going into the jaw
- o   phantom limb pain
- o   sciatica, if shooting pain

# Health Food Store Helpers for Frazzled Nerves

Although these are not for actual nerve damage, they are great for times when you feel "frazzled" or that your "nerves are shot."

**Kali phos,** a tissue salt or cell salt (see page 98), is great for times when your nerves feel depleted – say when you've been studying too much and especially from using the computer too much.

Get the 6x strength and dissolve two tablets in your mouth, as needed, maybe two or three times a day.

You may not find it in health food stores, but you can easily get it online, say from Homeopathic Educational Services, www.homeopathic.com.

Or you can get these two products, which include Kali phos: **Nerve Tonic by Hylands** is a blend of five cell salts, the ones that include phosphorus, because phosphorus is so important for the nervous system.

If your health food store doesn't have it, they should definitely have its sister remedy, **Calms Forte**, which includes the same minerals. It also contains a homeopathic dilution of several herbs which have been used for hundreds of years to calm the nerves and promote sound sleep.

## Story Time

I used to own a health food store near Harvard University, and Calms Forte was the most popular product in my store.

In this academic environment, where people were studying hard and not getting enough sleep, they would try Calms Forte and come back to buy several bottles for friends and family members, because they found it worked so well for frayed nerves, anxiety, and sleepless nights.

# Emotional First Aid

o  your teenage daughter's boyfriend just dumped her

o  your tween is the victim of mean, slanderous gossip being passed around the class via IM

o  your best friend's husband just left her for another woman

o  you just got the phone call you've been dreading – an elderly parent has passed away, or

o  another phone call you've been dreading – your teenager has had a car accident and is in the hospital

o  your boss just humiliated you in front of everyone at a staff meeting by blaming you for something to save face for himself.

We have a great concept in using these natural remedies – it's called **"hearing bad news"** –
like, someone gets sick (physically or emotionally) from "hearing bad news."

What do all these situations have in common?

**Sudden strong emotions,** whether grief or fear or shame or anger over injustice.

Natural remedies can help here too!
They can't change the situation –
but they can give you the inner strength, the poise and the presence of mind to deal with the situation in a mature way.

**IGNATIA** is your best friend in this situation – for sudden emotional upsets and stormy emotions in people of any age – it's especially great for teenagers!

"Sighing and sobbing" are the watchwords for this remedy – people show their tumultuous emotions by sobbing hysterically or heaving a sigh.

Sometimes, though, people react by going numb.
Instead of crying, they shut down.
They may feel like their brain freezes up and they can't think of what to do.

And they may feel so totally drained of energy that they can hardly move – that "just got run over by a truck" kind of totally flattened feeling.

You might wonder why someone might seem so emotionally flat in a very upsetting situation.

**GELSEMIUM** is your best friend for this kind of reaction.

We'll "make friends with Gelsemium" in the Flu chapter – because it's also our top remedy for the flu or any viral condition when the person feels totally flattened and drained of energy.

## Story Time

I was serving as a volunteer homeopath on a meditation retreat on Long Island. One young man asked for a remedy for what seemed to be the flu – quite odd on a sweltering August day! The typical flu symptoms were there: he felt absolutely lousy, he was totally drained of energy and even his eyelids were droopy.

I realized he needed Gelsemium but I thought that maybe he didn't actually have the flu – maybe there was something else going on. As we usually do when trying to find a remedy that matches well, I asked him what was the biggest stress in his life when he started to feel sick.

And as often happens, he said there was a big stress but he was sure it had nothing to do with getting the flu (which he was sure he had). He had gone into Manhattan and had not seen a hidden "No Parking/ Tow Zone" sign. His car was towed and it cost him several hundred dollars in cash to get it back – money he didn't really have.

Well, this is a great example of "hearing bad news"! First he went through the shock of thinking his car had been stolen. Then he found out that he had to fork over that much cash (when he didn't have that much in his account to withdraw).

To make matters worse, there was a storage fee for each day that he failed to pick up the car, so the cost kept going up and up while he tried to scrounge up the cash.

His body reacted to this series of "hearing bad news" as if it were punched down, like a boxer that gets punched down again before he can stagger to his feet. This kind of blow can make people react in a Gelsemium kind of way.

So that's why he seemed to have flu symptoms in August.

He perked right up after a dose of Gelsemium!

It's more common for people to get **OVER-emotional** rather than "NON-emotional" in a case of emotional upset – so let's make friends with Ignatia.

# Make Friends With IGNATIA

You already know three key words for Ignatia –

- o **sighing** (maybe from a feeling of a heavy weight on the chest)

- o **sobbing**

- o **stormy emotions**

Here's a couple more – then you know the whole remedy!

- o **psychosomatic symptoms** (physical symptoms that are really an expression of strong emotions)

- o **cramps and spasms** – muscle cramps or a cramping sensation

So let's put these concepts together and here's an overview of what you can use Ignatia for:

**emotional support** in a crisis

**insomnia** when upset, when "**rehearsing**" what happened the previous day ("I wish I said . . . ")

any **physical symptom** caused by stormy emotions, especially ones involving cramps or spasms:

- o spasmodic coughing

- o nausea/vomiting

- o lump in the throat (throat muscles cramped together)

- o back spasms or other muscle cramps

- o rectal spasms

- o colic in an infant – especially if the mom is upset!

# Now what?

"I've offered my friend some Ignatia and she says she wants to feel her emotions, she doesn't want to take a drug to numb herself to her grief."

This is an understandable reaction –
actually a praiseworthy reaction –
because too often in this society, people use all kinds of things to avoid feeling their feelings –

o   alcohol or drugs (whether prescription drugs or recreational drugs),

o   zoning out watching TV or immersing themselves in the internet, or

o   losing themselves in a fantasy world of gaming in which they've created another identity for themselves –
    one that can't be touched by grief.

When these forms of entertainment are used to avoid feeling grief or other strong emotion, several unhealthy things can happen.

o   The body may find an outlet for the strong emotions in the form of **physical illness** – we homeopaths see this all the time in our professional practice.

o   A lot of **life-energy is wasted** – a lot of life-energy is going into the emotion itself, and even more into suppressing the emotion – meaning that less is available for family, career, or creativity.

o   And it's **not a good role model for children** –
    kids have their little antennae out for parents who are upset or tense, and parents who numb themselves and avoid the problem are creating a not-helpful life-lesson for their kids.

EMOTIONAL FIRST AID o IGNATIA

So it's better to feel our painful feelings rather than numb ourselves.

Ignatia and other remedies don't numb the feelings, though.

They strengthen the core part of ourselves, the part that is processing the grief and coping with the difficult situation.

## Story Time

I remember I once had a client who missed her only son terribly – he had just left for college in another country, and it was dawning on her that he would probably never live at home again – so in some sense she had lost him, at least she had lost him as her little boy.

I offered her Ignatia and she refused it at first, saying she wanted to feel her feelings.

She was having a hard time functioning, she was crying so much, and – a sure clue to Ignatia – also sighing heavily.

Finally she took it, and was very pleased with the results.

She reported, "I can grieve without sobbing and I can feel my feelings without getting hysterical."

**Hysterical** is a great keyword for Ignatia!

# Health Food Store Helpers for Emotional First Aid

**Rescue Remedy** is also great for emotional upsets –
we made friends with Rescue Remedy in the first chapter.

I recommend that every home medicine chest have
Rescue Remedy on hand along with the other remedies
recommended in this book – because different things work
for different people.

You'll probably find at least one person in your family, or at
least one situation, where Rescue Remedy works better than
the "pellet remedies" in your kit.

In a good health food store, you're likely to find other things
that can help – perhaps a **guided meditation CD** or a
**yoga relaxation video.**

If you practice yoga and/or meditation on a regular basis,
you'll find yourself better prepared for the emotional ups and
downs of life.

Your yoga and meditation techniques will work better in
an emergency if you've already "strengthened your inner
muscles" by practicing them on a daily basis.

See Support Your Body's Healing Energy, page 120,
for some resources for learning them.

Here's another tip: simply **taking some deep breaths** can
help you calm down. You know how, when you get anxious,
your chest tightens up and your breathing gets shallow?
It works the other way around, too! Make yourself breathe
deeply, and you'll feel calmer.

# Quick Tip: If It Has an Alcohol Base

Rescue Remedy usually comes in a little bottle with a dropper tip – and usually you give it by putting a few drops on someone's tongue.

It's in an alcohol base, though, so this might not be ideal.

There's not enough alcohol to get you tipsy (just a few drops) but it might burn your tongue a little, kids may not like the taste, or you may have a religious or personal reason to avoid alcohol.

To overcome the taste or burning sensation
you can dissolve a few drops in a little water
and drink it that way.

**To totally avoid ingesting any alcohol,**
rub it (or the water solution) on temples,
inside of wrists, anywhere the skin is thin.


Homeopathic remedies have no alcohol –
so no problem!
they come in the form of tiny sugar pellets.


Herbal extracts like Echinacea are usually alcohol-based. You can often order a non-alcohol, glycerine-based form instead.

Or drive off the alcohol from an herbal extract by stirring it into hot water, like hot herbal tea.

# Drippy with a Cold

Do you have –

- o  your nose dripping like a faucet, like water drip-drip-drip, going through boxes of Kleenex?
- o  OR rattly yellow mucus?
- o  OR thick sticky, stringy mucus / greenish boogers?

Most people go through several phases with colds.

Usually the discharge starts off watery, ends up thick like rubber cement, and goes through a phase inbetween, when its consistency is more creamy or pudding-like.

The watery phase and the booger phase are the easiest to find remedies for:

**Watery** – either Arsenicum or Allium cepa.

**Arsenicum** – the most common in my practice, try it first

**Allium cepa** ("SEE-puh") – if there's an itchy nose, or red raw skin under the nose, a "red mustache"

## Thick and sticky –

There's really just one best remedy for this phase, **Kali bic** (sounds like "bick", we say "When mucus sticks, use Kali bic!") like when you blow your nose or cough up phlegm, and there's a long string of mucus to your mouth or nose – yuck!

**Kali bic** covers thick, sticky mucus anywhere in the body –

- o   in the nose

- o   in the sinuses

- o   in the ears, when you have to pop your ears,
     like in a plane but this time it's to clear the mucus

- o   mucus you can't get up from your lungs

Because the mucus is so sticky, it's hard to dislodge it – so you'll probably need to make the remedy stronger by putting it in water (see the Quick Tips on the next two pages).

The middle phase of a cold with medium thick rattly mucus has several possible remedies.

Try **Hepar sulph**, especially if the person is sensitive to cold and drafts and/or is irritable.

If Hepar sulph does not work, you'll need one of the more advanced books on pages 114–118.

You might want to master the simple situations in this book first – before you tackle a more complicated one where there are many remedies that might work.

# Quick Tip:
# Making the Remedies Stronger

Sometimes you need to make the remedy stronger –

o  because of the **situation** (like when you're flattened by the flu, or bleeding heavily and waiting for the ambulance)

o  or the **nature of the symptom** is hard to budge, like the thick sticky mucus of Kali bic

o  or the **person tends to be a slow responder** – you'll find this out by experience as you treat more family members and friends – some people usually feel remedies working as soon as they touch their mouth, while other people (like me! I'm slow when it comes to remedy reactions!) need a *lot* before they notice anything. In my experience, women tend to be more sensitive to the effect of the remedies, which might be why women tend to be more open-minded!

o  or there's something that **keeps triggering the condition** you're treating – let's say you're sick from getting soaked and chilled – normally you would get warm and dry, but what if you're out camping and the cold rain is relentless? (I hope you bring your remedies with you!)

To make the remedies stronger, you can

o  put them **in water** (see next page)

o  give them **more frequently** – the frequency of the dose is more important than the number of pellets in each dose. Remember the remedy is trying to teach your body something.

47

If you're trying to learn a song, you'll learn better from having one person sing it to you over and over (that's like repeating the remedy), than from having a lot of people sing it just once (which is like taking a lot of pellets in a single dose).

Taking a lot of pellets at once is only a little stronger than taking a few – it just wastes the pellets.

o   If you or someone in your family consistently need remedies stronger, you can get them in a **higher potency** (strength). The most commonly available higher potency is 200c – but that's a LOT stronger! I don't recommend it for home use, especially for beginners. Natural Health Supply has the remedies in a 100c potency – a more natural next step above the 30c. But please always start with the 30c in your kit before trying a higher potency. You'll be surprised at how much it can do.

# Quick Tip: Hypersensitives

Occasionally we come across someone who is sensitive
to everything – to medications, vitamins, and all kinds of
chemicals and fumes – and to every homeopathic remedy
you give them. These people are called "hypersensitives"
and you know who you are!

For hypersensitives, use a 6c potency, much milder than the
30c standard potency for self care.

Health food stores don't usually carry this mild potency. You
can order a First Aid Emergency Kit from Natural Health
Supply (see page 2) in a 6c strength.

When I teach a class of 20 to 30 people, usually there might
be one person who needs to order a 6c kit.

# Quick Tip: Giving Remedies in Water

Dissolving a couple of pellets in about a half cup of water, and taking it sip by sip, can make the remedies **stronger**!

Doesn't make any sense, does it?

The remedies are more dilute – how can they be stronger?

But the strength of the remedies is not based on the "stuff" in them – they work by giving your body a message, **information** about how to heal.
(See How the Remedies Work, page 110.)

When you dilute them in a small amount of water and stir really, really well, all of the water takes on the properties of the remedy pellet.

Each sip is like a great big pellet – it touches a much bigger area. If you **swish it like mouthwash** before swallowing, it will touch even more and can act even stronger.

We don't know exactly how the information is transmitted – but we know it happens because of the effect that it has – and we've found from experience that diluting in a little water makes the remedy stronger.

To make it even stronger – if you're not getting the results you expect and you're confident it's the right remedy – then you can **succuss the remedy**. You'll need to have it in a small bottle rather than a glass. Hold the bottle with one hand and whack it firmly against the palm of the opposite hand. (You can use a resilient surface like a mouse pad if your hand hurts.) This has the effect of energizing the remedy. You can succuss it ten times between sips.

# Health Food Store Helpers for Colds

Extra vitamin C – my own favorite is **Emergen-C**, which combines vitamin C with electrolyte minerals, each one enhancing the absorption of the other. It comes in little foil packets that fizz up when you add it to water.

I like to add the juice of half a lemon to a glass of water with raspberry-flavored Emergen-C – delicious!

It reminds me of a raspberry-lime rickey, one of the treats of my childhood.

**Immune boosting herbs** like echinacea, astragalus, andrographis – your health food store will have lots of information and suggestions about their favorite formula.

Remember that if you take an herb like this year round, it will lose its "oomph" because your body will get used to it. Save it for when you really need it – when you get run down or you're actually sick.

**Elderberry - honey syrup** – elderberry is a delicious berry that has antiviral activity, as does honey.

The combination is great when you're sick – take it by the spoonful, especially good for coughs. Kids love it!

# Making Friends With ARSENICUM

Okay, let's get it over with – how can you use a poison as a medicine?
It's totally **safe because there's "nothing in it"** –
not a single molecule of arsenic.

## So how can it work?
It's giving your body's healing energy the information it needs. For a longer explanation, see <u>How the Remedies Work</u>, page 110.
Your body *knows* how to be healthy –
it just gets thrown off base by different blows or shocks to the system, which can be physical or emotional.

The remedy gives the body information that reminds it of its natural healthy state. It's like calling in the piano tuner when your piano is out of tune. You wouldn't start with a hammer and saw, would you?

Anyway, getting back to Arsenicum, it will become one of your BEST remedy friends!

Here are your key concepts for Arsenicum:

o **anxious and fretful** about survival issues like health, money, having a roof over your head

o **extreme exhaustion** "out of proportion" (like, why would someone need to stay in bed for five days with a cold?)

o **burning** sensation

o **worse after midnight** (including insomnia)

Once you know that, you can use it for so many things:

- o acute anxiety
- o conjunctivitis
- o coughs
- o diarrhea, travelers' diarrhea
- o first stage of a cold
- o food poisoning
- o flu

- o hay fever
- o headaches
- o insomnia
- o mouth sores
- o nausea and vomiting
- o shingles
- o sore throats.

Of coure, you should also take these early warning symptoms as a sign that you need to slow down and take care of yourself. This is especially true for moms who tend to take care of everyone else first. But if you get sick, who will take care of them?

So be sure to get enough rest, eat nutrient-dense food, and avoid sugar and coffee especially when you are feeling rundown.

Plus this is a great time to take your immune herbs that you got at your local health food store!

What if you were a Peace Corps volunteer in a remote African village, teaching people hygiene to prevent cholera, and you were projecting images of people with cholera, using a laptop and a lightbox?

Anyone unfamiliar with the technology might run out of the hut, afraid of catching cholera!

But you would say, "There is no cholera there. Just the image. Just information that helps us to treat cholera."

Same deal with remedies. Just healing information.

# Now what?

"My nose isn't dripping any more – but my cold isn't gone – now the mucus is thicker."

Sometimes when we give a remedy right away, we can nip a cold in the bud and make it totally go away.

Sometimes, though, the best we can do is to speed the body through its natural progression of symptoms.

Let's say when you get a cold, you have a drippy watery nose and you're sneezing a lot for the first two or three days. Then you have rattly soft-thick mucus for another few days, ending up with lingering thick stringy mucus. The whole thing takes 7 to 10 days.

If you take a remedy the first day, you may find that you're already in the second phase the next day (needing another remedy) and in the last phase the third day (needing Kali bic) and the whole thing is over with in three days.

Success! You did a great job.

This is one of the ways the remedies can work for you. You just saved yourself a week of feeling miserable!

Make a note (yes, it's a good idea to keep a notebook) of what remedy you used first – the one that shifted the situation. Note what your symptoms were.

Next time you have those symptoms, take your first remedy right away, and maybe you'll be able to avert the cold instead of speeding it up.

# Droopy with the Flu

There are lots of remedies in your kit that might work for the flu. We'll keep it simple for now and just cover the most common ones.

You might as well try a remedy – conventional medicine has no treatment for flu except bed rest, and people are likely to be sick for several weeks with the flu.

Some day, we hope that public health officials will embrace the solution to flu epidemics that homeopaths wholeheartedly offer for the public good. The Spanish flu pandemic of 1918, the first swine flu, killed tens of millions of people worldwide **except those treated with homeopathy**, of whom only 1% died.

We have the same remedies today and are eager to offer them! They are safe and incredibly inexpensive – a whole community can be treated for a few dollars. We are only waiting to be asked!

These remedies are harmless at worst – and at best, in our experience, they can **shorten the flu** to a day or a few days, or even **avert it altogether.**

**Gelsemium** – your friend from the "Emotional First Aid" chapter – is our top favorite for the flu and other viral conditions.

You can recognize someone who needs it – drooping eyelids, so tired they can't get out of bed, they have fever and chills, and they feel apathetic, unlike our next contender . . .

**Arsenicum** – your friend from the Colds chapter – is really similar to the Gelsemium picture, with extreme tiredness, but likely to be anxious and fretful, restless and uncomfortable in bed even though they're exhausted. They are especially likely to be awake and restless between midnight and 2 am, which is their worst time. They are likely to have a sore throat and a drippy watery nasal discharge.

They might also have digestive symptoms, but a more likely remedy for a flu with digestive symptoms is . . .

**Nux vomica.** Doesn't the name just sound like it's for vomiting? Big clue – it's a great remedy for the digestive system from beginning (heartburn) to end (hemorrhoids)! Use it for the flu when the person has the chills and is really sensitive to noise, to being disturbed (they are really irritable!) or to the slightest draft of cold air that creeps in under the covers, where they will stay all bundled up.

One other remedy you already know – **Arnica** – for flu when the person feels sore and bruised. Honestly, not a very common flu remedy, but you have it in your kit – use it if the symptoms match!

There are lots of other possible remedies for flu. If none of these four remedies work, it's time for the more advanced books on pages 114–118.

# Health Food Store Helpers for Flu

For prevention – Oscillococcinum – call it "**Oscillo**" for short – is available these days in every health food store and many drugstores. The top selling flu remedy in France, it also works great for prevention. You don't need the whole tube, though, just a few pellets.

**Influenzinum** – may be a little harder to find in stores but you can usually get it from Homeopathic Educational Services, www.homeopathic.com, and Washington Homeopathics, www.homeopathyworks.com.

Usually we use a 9c (low potency) for prevention and 30c for treating the flu.

Sometimes this works better than "Oscillo". It may depend on the person, or maybe on the flu virus in a particular year. So it's worthwhile having both on hand.

**Dosage:** when the flu season starts, take either remedy once a week for four weeks, then once a month for the remainder of the flu season.

If you are directly and closely exposed to someone with the flu, in your family or at work, take a dose every day that the person is breathing on you.

Also the immune boosters mentioned in "Health Food Store Helpers for Colds" are important for the flu too.

# Quick Tip: "Nip It in the Bud"

In addition to the helpers listed for colds, we recommend keeping the cell salt **Ferrum phos** on hand. Your local health food store may carry cell salts (there are 12 of them and they may also be called tissue salts, see page 98). They will come in a little jar with 6x or 12x after their name (not in a tube labeled 30c).

Parents usually know when their kids are about to get sick – you know that look they get

- o   when they are under the weather
- o   listless, with no appetite
- o   no interest in things they usually enjoy
- o   maybe with a slight fever, but no real symptoms yet

and your parents' intuition tells you your child will probably be sick the next day.

You probably know the warning signs for yourself –

- o   you may feel rundown
- o   or get that funny scratchy vibration in the back of your throat that means sickness is trying to come in
- o   or – you know your own symptoms.

That's the perfect time for Ferrum phos!

Suck on two tablets, three times a day.
Kids love them – they taste sweet.

Of coure, you should also take these early warning symptoms as a sign that you need to slow down and take care of yourself. This is especially true for moms who tend to take care of everyone else first. But if you get sick, who will take care of them?

So be sure to get enough rest, eat nutrient-dense food, and avoid sugar and coffee especially when you are feeling rundown.

Plus this is a great time to take your immune herbs that you got at your local health food store!

# Making Friends with GELSEMIUM

This is our top remedy for flu and many viral conditions; also – remember the Emotional First Aid chapter – a great remedy for "hearing bad news" when the person reacts with emotional shutdown.

Here are your key concepts:

- o **dizzy, drowsy, droopy, dopy**

- o **anticipation anxiety** with diarrhea

- o **"hearing bad news"** and reacting with

- o **emotional numbness**

So here are LOTS of ways to use Gelsemium!

- o anxiety before the dentist
- o anxiety before the vet – for pets!
- o diarrhea
- o exam anxiety
- o fever and chills

- o flu
- o hayfever
- o insomnia
- o stage fright
- o vertigo

# Now what?

"I gave my child a dose of the remedy and he fell asleep in my arms. Help! Did I just drug my child?"

No, this means you did a great job!
Congratulations!

You gave the perfect remedy – well, maybe just a tiny bit too much of it.

If someone gets sleepy after a homeopathic remedy, it means her healing energy is going to work doing some deep healing.

It's like this.

Imagine you have a little shop and you want to do some renovations – refinish the floor, freshen up the paint, rearrange the displays.

You put a sign on the door "Closed for renovations" because you can't handle customers at the same time.

In a day or two you reopen – with your shop transformed, more beautiful than ever.

Your body's healing energy does something like that when you give it a remedy.

Remember that the remedy is actually "operating instructions" or a kind of blueprint to teach the body's healing energy how to fix things.

If it's a little too strong, the body wants to hurry up and fix everything quickly – so it has to "close the store for business" for a few hours while it goes to work.

It's not at all like drowsiness as a side effect of a medication. You can tell because it only happens in the beginning, if at all – and it leaves you feeling much better than before the remedy.

Honestly, this doesn't usually happen – but if it does, it's great.

If your child gets sleepy after a dose, just let him sleep and he's likely to be much better when he wakes up – in fact he may not even need any more of the remedy.

# Story Time

True story – in the early days of my practice, I was still learning what instructions I needed to give along with the remedy.

A mom brought her little boy to see me – he had a chronic cough and sometimes asthma attacks. Homeopathy is great for asthma, by the way – a professional homeopath can help you overcome it for good.

In this case, the boy had a little cough when his mom brought him to see me. I gave her the specific remedy that matched his particular cough symptoms, with instructions to give it hourly until he got better, then to stop.

I gave her a standard 30c strength, the one carried in health food stores, but the boy was unusually sensitive to homeopathy, as it turned out, and would have done better with a milder dose.

He got worse (had a boomerang experience, an "aggravation" as we call it) right from the first dose. He started coughng more, and since he wasn't getting better, the mom kept giving it – until, after three doses, he fell asleep.

She called to see if she should wake him up for his next dose – which is something we might do with conventional medicine, but not with these natural remedies, because sleeping means healing.

She explained the situation and I realized I forgot an important part of the instructions – that if he got worse right away, she should also stop.

No harm, I told her – just let him sleep, and when he wakes up, his cough will be gone.

I was confident saying that, because I knew what had happened – he got the right healing remedy (if it were the wrong remedy for him, he most likely would not have reacted at all) and he got more than enough to make the cough go away.

Sure enough, his mom called a few hours later – it worked out just as I told her it would!

# Sick to Your Stomach?

o    Your child says "Mommy, my tummy hurts, I don't
     want to go to school" (but as soon as you let her
     stay home and cuddle with you, she suddenly feels
     better!)

o    You might have eaten something bad and now
     you're nauseous, about to throw up

o    or your child has a stomach bug and has been
     throwing up every 15 minutes all night

A couple of great remedies for gastrointestinal distress cover
a lot of situations.

The main question to ask, if the person in question is a child
– is she really, really sick, or is her tummy upset maybe an
excuse for special attention?

**Pulsatilla** is our top remedy for children's acute illnesses in
general – especially if the child tends to be cuddly when well
and even clingier when sick. She may want to climb on your
lap and snuggle and want extra attention and reassurance –
"Mommy, do you love me?" I mean, she may honestly feel
sick – but when mom's special attention is her best medicine,
Pulsatilla can speed up the cure.

In other situations (including for kids when they're not
showing these symptoms) our favorite remedy is **Nux vomica.**

If food poisoning is involved, think first of **Arsenicum**.
People who need Arsenicum are likely to be anxious and

restless, and to have burning pains. People who need Nux vomica are likely to be irritable with spasmodic cramping.

Remember that throwing up can be the body's way to protect itself against, say, spoiled food. If you give a remedy and the person throws up right away, maybe the remedy gave the body extra strength to do what it needed to do anyway.

## Story Time

This happened to me after drinking a bottle of the fermented health drink Kombucha. It's usually one of my favorite things, but maybe this bottle had not been properly prepared . . . anyway, I felt nauseous as soon as I drank it. I took some Nux vomica and instantly threw up.

I knew this must be a positive effect of Nux because

... it's the first time in 50 years that I've thrown up (so it wasn't a coincidence), and ...

... I never aggravate on remedies (my symptoms never intensify because the remedy is too strong)

So I concluded that my body, in its wisdom, used the information from the dose of Nux to speed up what it was trying to do anyway.

The takeaway message here is that homeopathy does not **suppress symptoms** i.e. force symptoms to disappear while leaving the underlying problem untouched.

Suppressing symptoms is dangerous because the underlying problem has to find another way to vent itself – usually a more destructive way than before.

Suppressing the body's symptoms is like blocking the little jiggler valve on top of a pressure cooker. Eventually it will explode! and the body will find new symptoms as an outlet.

# Make Friends with NUX VOMICA

Nux covers problems in the digestive tract, from heartburn to hemorrhoids, plus several others to boot!

Here are your key concepts for Nux vomica:

- o **digestive** problems

- o **cramps** and cramping pain

- o **worse from overindulging** in rich/fatty food, junk food, spicy food, alcohol

- o **irritable**

- o **chilly** – if they are under the covers, even a tiny crack that lets a draft in is unbearable

So here are a wide range of **digestive conditions** Nux can help with, IF the symptoms match:

| | |
|---|---|
| o cramping pains in abdomen | o heartburn |
| o constipation | o hemorrhoids |
| o diarrhea | o nausea |
| o acute gallbladder attack | o vomiting |
| o hangovers | o stomach cramps |

plus more that are not digestive symptoms:

| | |
|---|---|
| o back pain | o insomnia, waking at 3 a.m. |
| o bladder infection | o lower back pain |
| o colds | o menstrual cramps |
| o coughs | o muscle cramps, in general |
| o flu | o passing kidney stones |
| o hayfever | |

Isn't it amazing how many things you can treat with one little tube of a remedy?

It won't work if the symptoms don't match – there are other remedies for each of these conditions – but in general there's no harm in trying.

The big exception is if you are hypersensitive – if you tend to overreact to everything, you'll probably overreact to homeopathy, and you need to be cautious about experimenting!

## Story Time

My friends' black Lab is always getting into everything – garbage, roadkill, you name it. The raunchier the better!

Nux vomica is this dog's best friend.

Yes, remedies work just as well for animals as they do for people.

To give a remedy to an animal, you can put a pellet inside its lip or stir it into the water bowl.

# Now what?

"I've given three doses of the remedy and there's no change."

You have to use your common sense here.

**Is it a situation that might actually change after three doses?**
Let's say you have a broken bone. A remedy won't fix that in three doses.
It's still worth giving **Symphytum**, our remedy for healing fractures. Symphytum can help the healing take only half as long – but broken bones take weeks to mend.
Symphytum is really the only choice for broken bones so don't second-guess yourself, just keep taking it (along with its Best Remedy Friend Calc phos 6x – see page 98).

Or – **if it's something that actually could change,**
maybe you need to try a different remedy.

Nausea is a great example of that. If someone is feeling nauseous, and you give them the right remedy, they could feel better right away.

If you've given three doses over several hours and the person is still just as nauseous, it's time to try a different remedy.

Another possibility – **maybe the remedy isn't strong enough.**

As you get experience treating yourself and your loved ones, you'll find that different people respond to different strengths and different ways of giving the remedies.

Keep notes in a special notebook.

You may find that one family member is very sensitive – what we call a "hypersensitive" – and is so reactive to homeopathy that she can feel a good remedy working right away.

If she doesn't feel anything from the first dose, you need to find a better remedy for her.

You may find that another family member tends to be a slow responder and to need a lot of the remedy. Maybe he tends to need the remedy dissolved in water, taken with lots of stirring or shaking and frequent sips (described on page 48).

If this case, if he hasn't responded after three doses, you would still keep trying.

At some point you'll need to rethink your remedy choice.

This is something you'll learn by experience – and keeping notes will help a lot.

## Story Time

One of my first dramatic experiences with homeopathy was with my running buddy. (I've never had my own dramatic experience. Does that make you feel better? I know the remedies work for me, but I just can't *feel* them working!)

Anyway, we were driving to Fresh Pond for our Saturday morning run around the pond, and she said, "You know, I don't think I can do this. I've got my period and suddenly I'm getting really bad cramps."

We happened to be going past my health food store, so I stopped and got her some **Mag phos,** one of our favorite cramp remedies. We turned to drive home again, and she stopped at the next traffic light and looked at me in amazement.

"Is it possible it could have worked so fast?"

That was one of the experiences that made me want to study homeopathy!

# Quick Tip: Put Together a Travel Kit

You've probably noticed that several of these remedies would be great to have on hand while you're traveling. Here's a review, plus a couple more we haven't talked about yet:

○ **Arsenicum** for traveler's diarrhea

○ **Nux vomica** for upset stomachs from unfamiliar food

○ **Arnica – Calendula – Phosphorus,** the injury trio

○ **Carbo veg.** if you are going to a higher altitude where you may have difficulty breathing, because this remedy helps your body absorb oxygen more effectively. By the way, it's also great for intestinal gas!

○ **Cocculus** if you will be changing time zones, because this remedy helps your body adjust its internal clock. Take a few pellets before take-off and another few pellets when you land.

○ If Cocculus does not work for you, try **No Jet Lag**, which you can get in any health food store. I've taken a poll among hundreds of friends on international meditation retreats. Most people use No Jet Lag because it works for them. But if it doesn't, try Cocculus, which works better for me.
Also, if you bought a kit you already have Cocculus in your kit and chances are that it will work for you, as it has for almost everyone I've given it to.
In other words, either one is likely to work for most people.

# Stings and Hives

You can cover a lot of these problems with just one remedy – **APIS** – because using these natural remedies is based on symptoms, not diagnosis.

That means that if you or your child has

o   a **raised red bump** that looks **swollen**

o   maybe feels **warm**

o   maybe feels **burning** and/or **itchy**

o   in other words, **like a bee sting**

Apis is likely to work, whether it's from an insect bite or an allergic reaction.

If it doesn't, you're likely to need another remedy – time for one of the more advanced books on pages 114–118!

# Make Friends With APIS

Just to review, your key words for Apis are:

**swollen** . . . **red** . . . **warm** or **burning** . . . **itchy** . .
**looks like a bee sting**.

Look at how many different ways Apis can be used!

o   allergic reactions

o   bee stings

o   bladder infections

o   canker sores

o   chicken pox

o   conjunctivitis

o   fever

o   herpes

o   hives

o   insect bites

o   menstrual cramps

o   poison ivy

o   poison oak

o   rashes

o   tonsillitis

o   urine retention in newborns

Here are a couple more:

a sore throat with a **swollen uvula**
(the little thing that hangs down in the back of your throat

**water retention** even when there's no redness, burning or
itching – like when your rings don't fit before your period,
or when your ankles swell on the plane. (You know how you
can't get your shoes back on when the plane is about to
land?)

# Story Time

One of my homeopathy students, Shirley Moore, uses homeopathic remedies in her wonderful clinic that saves dogs from shelters and prepares them for adoption. She teaches the use of simple remedies, like those in this book, to her volunteers and to the families adopting her dogs.

Here is one story from Shirley's clinic, in her own words:

"A ten week old Lab pup was showing symptoms of a bee sting at her foster home and she had all the signs of an allergic reaction. In the short drive over to my house, the puppy's eyes became swollen shut and her face was swollen to at least twice its normal size. She was lethargic and panting. The plan was to take her to an emergency vet hospital but she was in such bad shape, I was afraid she would die on the way.

"So I gave her the remedy Apis and the swelling went down in five short minutes! If there weren't witnesses in the room, I wouldn't have believed my eyes. This simple remedy saved the puppy's life."

To read more about Shirley's wonderful work with dogs, please see the second part of this series. Shirley has contributed a whole section on her simple techniques for rescuring dogs with homeopathy!

# Health Food Store Helper for Stings and Hives

**Seven Cream** is an amazing skin cream for lots of itchy and/ or dry skin conditions, including poison ivy, insect bites, even eczema and psoriasis.
My own clients have reported great results for almost all of these conditions.

It's not expected to cure longterm conditions, but it can give you great relief while you're seeking professional help from a naturopath or homeopath.

If your local health food store doesn't have Seven Cream, recommend that they get it from www.natural-skin-health.com.

Or you can get it online from www.mirandacastro.com.

It's one of those things that you might as well get now, before you need it, because you'll definitely use it at some point, and you'll be glad you did.

# Quick Tips: Splinters and Fungal Nails

As long as we're talking about skin stuff, here are just a couple of favorite more favorite tips:

**Thuja** can be used as a toenail dip for fungus under the nails. Dissolve a pellet in about half a cup of water (you may have to crush it to dissolve it) and put it in a clean container like an old deli container. Soak you toenails in it for ten minutes twice a day. My clients have told me they can see clean pink nails growing out within the first week!

**Silica** can push out anything embedded under the skin, like a splinter, a shard of glass, shrapnel, or all the little bits of gravel that get embedded in your kid's knee when he falls off his bike. One dose is often enough, but you can safely give a dose twice a day until the object works it's way out.

**Silicea** (the cell salt version) strengthens brittle hair and nails, and also helps people with fragile skin that is slow to heal.

## Story Time

A dear friend and fellow homeopath tells of giving Silica to a little girl who had fallen onto broken glass, and even after her mother picked out what she could, the little girl's hand was still filled with tiny fragments.

After the dose of Silica, at first it felt like a whole crop of little stiff hairs all over the girl's hand. Then the tiny shards of glass emerged and fell out!

ᘒ

I had a similar experience giving Silica to a friend who had stepped on a sea urchin, and the thin bony spines were embedded in her foot. A dose of Silica pushed them to the surface so that they were easy to remove.

# Sprains, Strains and Creaky Joints

These conditions have two top remedies which are easy to distinguish.
One or the other is likely to help a lot of joint pain.

As always, if neither one helps, it means a different remedy is needed. There are actually lots of possible remedies and you'll learn about them in the advanced books on pages 114–118.

If the joint pain is recent – say from a sprained ankle – you can relieve the pain and speed up the healing with natural remedies.
If the joint pain is chronic – say from arthritis or fibromyalgia – you can get temporary relief to tide you over while seeking professional help from a homeopath or naturopath.

In other words, don't expect to cure longstanding joint problems with these home remedies – but they are safe to try and may provide you with good short-term relief.

**Rhus tox** – our most common remedy for sprains, strains and joint pains – is called the "rusty gate remedy".
People who need it feel stiff and need to limber up.
They may wake up in the morning feeling stiff and may have to spend a few minutes doing stretching exercises.

**Bryonia** – the second most common remedy – has the opposite quality so it's easy to tell them apart.
People who need Bryonia feel more pain from the slightest movement.
So they do what we call 'guarding' or 'splinting' – they try to hold the body part absolutely still to avoid more pain.

# Make friends with RHUS TOX

Rhus tox works for lots more than just joint pain!

Remember these three concepts and then you'll get a handle on all of its uses:

o **"rusty gate"** – stiff at first, need to limber up

o feel better from **warmth, hot water**

o **blisters that look like poison ivy**
(not surprisingly, because it's actually made from a highly dilute extract of poison ivy –
safe because there are no molecules left)

So here are things you can use it for, if the Rhus tox themes are present:

| | |
|---|---|
| o back pain | o joint pain |
| o chicken pox | o shingles |
| o fever blisters, cold sores | o sore throats |
| o flu with cold sores | o sprains and strains |
| o impetigo | o whiplash |

One odd thing that doesn't fit with the others:

o hoarseness when the voice breaks and gives out

maybe because the vocal cords are muscles that can get strained too!

# friends with BRYONIA

**"...s dry"** is a key concept for Bryonia.
People who need it tend to have dry mucous membranes (mouth, colon) and they tend to need a lot of water.

They're really thirsty but the slightest movement may hurt – so once they start drinking they tend to drink a lot to get it over with quickly!

Bryonia is especially good for areas that provide lubrication between body parts – like where the moveable parts of joints rub together, or where the lungs rub against the chest when you breathe.

When those areas dry out, **it hurts to move**!

So for example, the person may have a dry cough that is so painful, they hold their ribs to try to keep their chest from moving when they have to cough.

One more thing – people who need it tend to be irritable and want to be left alone – it's been called the **"grouchy bear in the cave"** remedy.

Here are some ways you can use Bryonia:

- o  arthritis
- o  broken bones (for the pain)
- o  constipation with dry stool
- o  coughs (painful, dry)

- o  fractures
- o  headaches
- o  mastitis
- o  sprains and strains

You can also use it for appendicitis while on the way to the hospital – it's our most common remedy. In the days before 911, the old homeopaths used to *cure* appendicitis with it.

# Health Food Store Helpers

Miranda Castro's **Joint Cream** is absolutely amazing, in my experience and in that of my clients and students.
It can provide quick relief – sometimes even in cases of longstanding joint pain.

If your local health food store doesn't carry it yet, please suggest it to them.

In the meantime you can get it online from www.mirandacastro.com.

And by the way, you can see Miranda give a wonderful short description of joint pain and back pain remedies on YouTube, on GreenHealingTV!

## Story Time

My chiropractor friend wrenched her right thumb in a skiing accident, and it took weeks to heal. For anyone who works with her hands, that's a long time! Even Arnica was not doing the job.

She said Joint Cream was what really did the trick. After four days of Joint Cream, her thumb was much better.

That's high praise coming from a chiropractor – she really knows her joints!

# Now what?

"I gave the remedy and I'm not feeling better or worse –
just different – my symptoms changed!"

Occasionally the wrong remedy will stimulate the body's
healing energy to produce a new symptom, one that is a clue
to the right remedy.

It's as though giving a remedy opens a direct line of
communication to the body's healing energy.

I can't explain how this works – but I can tell you that it
does work, and that I've seen it happen many times in my
practice. Actually the best way to explain it is with a story.

## Story Time

A client who was new to homeopathy and very enthusiastic was giving her two-year-old daughter Arsenicum for a cold, following my instructions perfectly. Her daughter was sneezing a lot, typical for Arsenicum, and had the classic watery discharge.

After three doses, her daughter was no better – in fact she was worse. She had developed some new symptoms. Her cheeks and the skin under her nose were red and chapped.

This told me that she needed Allium cepa, the other great remedy for sneezing with lots of watery discharge. It can be a little hard to tell which one people need, because the symptoms are so similar, including the "red mustache" under the nose – really typical for Allium cepa, but Arsenicum patients can need it too.

The red chapped cheeks were a dead giveaway for Allium cepa, though, and she got better right away with Allium cepa.

# Teething

We'll just do one more condition, because it's so easy to distinguish between two of the top remedies, and because the results are so dramatic if you find one that works.

**Pulsatilla** is our top remedy for ailments for small children in general, when the child is sweet, clingy, cuddly, needy, demanding of attention and affection, and easily changing from tears to smiles when comforted ("like April weather, rainshowers to sunshine", our classic texts would say).

When this type of child is in pain from teething, they are likely to be whiny, to want mom to hold them, and to burrow their head in mom's chest.

These are also the kids who want to sleep in mommy and daddy's bed longer than other kids!

When you give these kids Pulsatilla for teething – or any other condition that calls for it – you're likely to see "positive side effects" like a three year old who suddenly announces he's ready to use the potty or who wants to go to daycare instead of clinging to mom's leg like a little barnacle.

It's not our top remedy for teething, though – that honor goes to **Chamomilla**, for a child who is absolutely screaming with pain which turns her into a little monster of insatiable demands.

This child will demand one thing after another – no sooner do you hand it to her than she hurls it to the floor and screams for something else. No matter how hard you try to please her, she is always dissatisfied – because she wants something else.

The old masters of homeopathy would say, "You want to hug a Pulsatilla child and spank a Chamomilla child."

Just give Chamomilla, though, and it will relieve the teething pain and restore the child to her normal wonderful self!

By the way, if you want to see Miranda Castro do a really funny impersonation of these two types, check out our YouTube channel, GreenHealingTV, and look for Miranda's Teething video. Fun!

Remember, though, remedies may not work if they don't match the particular person. That's the tricky thing about these remedies. They are not drugs. They are information packets, giving your body the information it needs. If a child is teething and not acting like a Pulsatilla or a Chamomilla child, her body probably wants the information from a different remedy.

Please don't get overwhelmed with how much there is to know. Start small and keep it simple.

That's what this book is about. Maybe learn one remedy a month for the next year – doesn't that sound manageable? You can do so much with these simple remedies!

Then when you've mastered the simple remedies and basic situations in this book, you can move on to more complicated ones.

I've seen so many people who are new to homeopathy become frustrated because they totally fall in love with it and want to fix everything all at once. You can't! Just focus on all the good that you are doing. You're way ahead of the game just using these basic remedies!

# Make Friends With PULSATILLA

Pulsatilla is used based on the personality (sweet, clingy, cuddly, sometimes whiny and gently manipulative) and on the stage of life (infants and young children) as much as on the specific conditions.

Almost any health concern in a young child can be well treated with Pulsatilla if the personality matches as well as some well known typical symptoms:

o   craving **fresh air** and **gentle exercise** –
    maybe a walk or at least an open window

o   indigestion from **rich, fatty foods**

o   a tendency to refuse to drink ("**thirstless**"),
    even with a fever

It's especially appropriate for children who feel **abandoned**, whether because they are sent to daycare too early, or even because their birth was induced. Babies have their own idea of when it's time to come out.

The physical conditions covered can be

o   **infectious** like ear infections, conjunctivitis, colds, flu

o   **developmental** like teething and potty training

o   **gastrointestinal** like stomachache, diarrhea.

## Tip: Pulsatilla for Pets

nd kittens are often separated from their mothers and sent to their new homes because they are so cute at that young age. They may then bond to their new families and become extremely affectionate, "clinging" to their new "mother's" lap.

For this type of cat or dog, Pulsatilla is likely to be a wonderful remedy. Try it!

## Now what?

"My symptoms keep getting worse! What do I do?"

You have to think – would they have gotten worse anyway? Sometimes a situation is on its way to getting really intense, and you are slowing it down – that's good, you just need to keep going and make the remedy stronger.

Other times it's something that really should respond to homeopathy, and if it doesn't – time to try a different remedy.

## Story Time

One of my clients brought her three-and-a-half year old son to me in desperation – because he was about to be expelled from daycare! He was still not potty trained, and the daycare owners (a Russian mother and grandmother) believed children should be out of diapers by their first birthday.
They were putting their collective feet down about changing any more diapers for this boy.

He was a sweet boy, a "mama's boy," and fit the Pulsatilla profile. Also, he was certainly aware that his parents were making plans for the imminent birth of his little sister – clearly he was feeling edged out of his spot as his mom's special darling.

He seemed to have gotten the message that his mom really wanted another baby, and on some level he seemed to be trying to be more "babyish" to secure her attention – reverting to thumbsucking, asking for a bottle and so forth.

Pulsatilla can be great at moving kids appropriately through the developmental stages. I gave him one dose of Pulsatilla and he announced to his mother, "I'm a big boy now. I want to use the potty!" and that was the end of diapers for him, to his mother's enormous relief. It was just in time – before the next little one arrived to create the next avalanche of diapers!

## Story Time

A friend had a Schnauzer who was totally attached to her, always wanting to sit in her lap with his paws on her shoulders. He also liked to ride in the car with his nose out the window.

For years she worked at home, but then when she got a day job he started peeing on the rug while she was at work. Based on these hints, I suggested she give him Pulsatilla. I guessed that he was feeling abandoned and was "acting out" like a little kid acting babyish.

It worked!

# Health Food Store Helpers

If neither of these remedies matches your child's symptoms, or works for her teething pain, you can always use **Calc phos**, a cell salt or tissue salt (see page 98).

Actually you can use it alongside the remedies because it helps build strong bones and teeth, and it will help push out those little teeth.

The tablets are soft and dissolve almost on contact with the mouth.

If giving them to a small baby, you can dissolve one in a little water and dab it onto the lips and gums.

One tablet, or one dab of the water, three times a day or as needed.

These remedies are so gentle, they can be safely given as often as you need.

You can always use **Hyland's Teething Tablets** or **Teething Gel** – these are old favorites, and they were among the most popular products in my health food store.

They are a combination of several possible remedies for teething, which increases the chances that at least one of them will work.

## Story Time

I've heard many stories from the parents of my little clients about how much their children love taking homeopathic remedies. It's not unusual for a four- or five-year-old to have mastered the names of the remedies she usually needs and to ask for a remedy by name when she feels sick.

It's also not unusual for a toddler to toddle over to the cupboard where the medicines are stored and pat the cupboard door to indicate he wants a remedy.

Here's my favorite story, though.

The mother of a 10-month-old infant was already using Hyland's Teething Tablets when she brought her baby to see me for another issue. She mentioned that the baby seemed to have learned the sound of the pellets rattling in the tube.

He would be crying with teething pain, then hear the rattle of the pellets as she got out the tube.

Instantly cries would turn into a big smile as the baby kicked and waved with glee knowing that relief was on the way. This was before she even gave him a dose!

# Resource Section

Cell Salts (Tissue Salts) ........................................ 98

Safety Guidelines.................................................. 99

Partner With Your Doctor ................................... 104

Find a Doctor to Partner With ............................ 106

Find a Professional Homeopath.......................... 108

How the Remedies Work .................................... 110

What to Say to a Skeptic.................................... 112

Dive Deeper – Reference Materials..................... 114

Books to Enjoy Reading ...................................... 116

Books on Specific Topics ..................................... 118

Websites to Explore ............................................ 119

Support Your Body's Healing Energy ................... 120


About the Author ................................................ 123

Index of Remedies and Supplements.................. 125

Index of Conditions............................................. 126

# Cell Salts (Tissue Salts)

Cell salts or tissue salts (known in Europe as Schuessler salts) are a special type of homeopathic remedy made from twelve combinations of the most common minerals the body needs, like calcium, potassium and magnesium.

Minerals are hard for the body to absorb – think little rocks going through the digestive system. One way to use cell salts is simply to help minerals absorb better. For example, **Ferrum phos** is used for anemia, to help absorb iron better, and **Calc phos** is used for osteoporosis, to help absorb calcium better.

So in one way they are like mineral supplements, except that they are homeopathically "energized" for better absorption.

They can also have therapeutic benefits. For example, **Nat mur** (sodium chloride) helps "teach" the body where water belongs. It can balance things out whether an area is too dry, or if the person is retaining water – either way, something is out of whack with the water balance.
And **Ferrum phos** can be used to prevent colds and flu.

If a store has them, they will be on a shelf in a set of 12 near the homeopathic remedies. They will probably be labeled 6x (that's the strength; it doesn't mean to take them 6 times a day). Occasionally a store has them in the milder 12x potency.

A typical dosage is two pellets three times a day.

Cell salts are a great place to start learning homeopathy. The best source for more information is the DVD by Miranda Castro, **Gentle Little Souls: The 12 Fabulous Cell Salts,** available on her website, www.mirandacastro.com.

# Safety Guidelines

This is a guide, not a complete list.

Be safe and do not take chances.

When in doubt, call your doctor or 911.

Work with a doctor who knows you are using natural remedies, and who will help you know what's safe and what's not. Your doctor may have different rules than these.

**Consider the situation:** Use common sense.

o   If this is a condition for which you would normally call 911 or take the person to the ER, do that. You can give remedies on the way, or while waiting for the EMTs to arrive.

o   Do not delay seeking conventional medical assistance.

o   Once the person is under the care of the EMTs or hospital, do not give remedies unless the person requests it on the spot, or unless it's your own child (for legal reasons).

o   It's generally not advisable to treat someone else's child with non-conventional methods, even with the best of intentions and even in an emergency, without the express permission of the parents.

**Consider the condition:** Use common sense as to whether it's safe to use homeopathy and delay conventional treatment.

An excellent guide is Cummings and Ullman's *Everybody's Guide to Homeopathic Medicine*, which lists "Beyond Home Care" signs for many common conditions (guidelines for when you need to call the doctor or go to the hospital).

Here are some typical signs that you should seek conventional care urgently:

**Difficulty breathing** for any reason including if the person has been stung by a bee or inhaled something that can't be coughed up.

**Rapid breathing** should always be evaluated

o   keep in mind that children normally breathe faster than adults

o   and of course people normally breathe faster after exercise.

**Wheezing:** moderate or severe wheezing with difficulty breathing

Mental state: **confusion or lack of awareness** of surroundings in someone normally mentally healthy can indicate a severe infection or other serious condition

**Loss of consciousness** following head injury (or actually, for any reason)

**Fevers:** a fever of 101° in a child under six months;

o   in others, a fever of 103.5° or higher that does not respond within 6 hours to home care (giving remedies, bathing or sponging down with lukewarm water);

o   any fever that has lasted longer than 24 hours in children 6 to 24 months,

o   or longer than 72 hours in others.

**Loss of fluids:** prolonged fever or vomiting and/or diarrhea can lead to **dehydration:** a baby can become dehydrated in only 24 hours, older children and adults in just a couple of days; this may require IV fluids in the hospital.

**Seizures;** such as febrile seizures (during a fever in a small child) or after a head injury

**Vomiting** if severe and prolonged, especially after a head injury

**Eyes:** severe eye pain, injury to the eye,

- o chemical or foreign object in the eye;

- o loss of vision;

- o if light causes pain in the eye;

- o if the pupil is shaped irregularly or does not react to changes in light

**Bleeding:** unexplained bleeding from the mouth, nose or rectum, or bloody urine;

- o bleeding or fluid from nose or ears following head injury;

- o bleeding from a cut that won't stop

**Abdominal pain**: check for appendicitis: in the lower right part of the abdomen, press in with a finger firmly and let go; pain on releasing your finger ("rebound tenderness") is a strong indicator for appendicitis, which is a serious emergency

**Kidney pain** can indicate a kidney infection, a potentially very serious condition. This is especially likely if the person has recently had a urinary tract infection and now has lower back pain with a fever. Have the person lean over a chair and tap on the spot where the lowest rib attaches to the spine. Pain at that spot is probably kidney pain.

**Animal bites:** if from an unknown (possibly rabid) animal; or if red streaks start leading towards the heart.

**Rare, very dangerous conditions:** unlikely to happen but you should memorize these symptoms:

o Child who is leaning forward, drooling, can't swallow or talk, looks like throat is closed up (could be epiglottitis)

o Stiff neck with headache, fever, seizures (could be meningitis).

This is by no means a complete list!

Be safe. Please consult *Everybody's Guide* or call your doctor if in doubt.

## Story Time

I was on the volunteer medical team on a retreat in a tropical country, working with a homeopathic primary care physician.

Late one night we were summoned to the room of a woman who had been out in the sun all day and seemed severely dehydrated to the point of being delirious. Her roommate was concerned because she was lying in bed, too weak to get up, and she was babbling and not making any sense.

The physician was about to give her intravenous fluids which he had brought on the retreat for this purpose.

But we decided to try a homeopathic remedy first – **China** or **Cinchona** (same thing), well known in homeopathy for what we call "loss of vital fluids" whether through perspiration, vomiting, diarrhea or bleeding.

We gave her a dose of China, went to check on some other sick folks, and came back in half an hour.

We were amazed to find her sitting up in bed, bright eyed and perky, eating and joking around with her roommate! China had acted as well as the IV fluids would have, to restore her to health!

# Partner With Your Doctor

When treating your children, and especially babies, you want to be extra sure that you are doing it safely.

For example, if your child's fever starts to rise, you'll want to know how high the fever can go before you really do need to give a conventional medicine. There's no hard and fast rule – it depends on your child's overall demeanor.

You need to work with your doctor – so if you want to use natural remedies for home care, it's best to **find a doctor who is supportive.**

If they are not, they will automatically tell you to bring in anyone who is sick. But going to a doctor's office (or even worse, an emergency room) can expose you to worse contagion. Plus you can become overmedicalized, getting tests and drugs you do not need.

In particular, doctors often prescribe antibiotics even when the condition is viral (antibiotics won't work in this situation).

Doctors often say they feel pressure from patients to prescribe something. However, the Centers for Disease Control of the US government have asked doctors **not to prescribe unnecessary antibiotics** – because these contribute to the development of antibiotic-resistant bacteria, which is bad for our public health in general.

So there is government support for the practice of **not** treating common conditions with antibiotics if possible.

**You are doing your part for public health** by using natural remedies when it's safe to do so.

Ideally you would like to be able to work with your doctor and find out how long it's safe to treat a condition at home, or how high a fever can go or how long a cough can go on before the situation becomes urgent and you really have to go to the doctor or hospital.

If your doctor is overly skeptical or sarcastic, if your doctor makes fun of your efforts or makes you feel stupid, it is time to find another doctor.

Most doctors, though, are simply skeptical of something they are unfamiliar with.

While doctors in many other countries around the world are trained in these natural remedies or refer patients to their colleagues who are, here in America medical schools have only recently begun including some reference to natural healing.

In fact, the American Medical Association recently adopted a recommendation that doctors educate themselves about alternative practices.

You can do your part by telling your doctor about your good results with natural healing. The more doctors hear about this from their patients, the more comfortable they'll be with these modalities.

Your doctor may say these remedies are "unproven". See What to Say to a Skeptic on page 112.

In short, they often *do* have research behind them – and if not, "unproven" doesn't mean "they don't work." It simply means "not yet proven", usually for lack of research funds. These remedies have a 200-year track record of safe and effective use.

# Find a Doctor to Partner With

You need a primary care doctor who is supportive or at least open-minded about your use of natural remedies. Here are some ideas about how to find one. You may not need to find an MD to act as your PCP. If you are lucky, you can get a real nature-doctor – called a naturopath!

**Naturopaths** are health care professionals who go through years of training, like doctors, except they learn how to use natural remedies, herbs, vitamins and healthy food instead of drugs. In about 15 to 20 states, naturopaths can act as primary care physicians.

Check www.naturopathic.org, click on About Naturopathic Medicine then Licensure to see if they are licensed in your state.
If so, you can check the directory listing for your state on the same website.

If not, here are some other approaches.

You may find that **nurse practitioners** are more open-minded about natural methods than doctors are, because nurses' training tends to be more holistic.

In many states nurse practitioners can act as primary care providers. You may also find that women and younger doctors/nurse practitioners, in general, are more open-minded (although we also hear of grandmother-age practitioners who fondly remember the home remedies of their youth).

Here's what you probably *don't* need:
a physician listed as a practitioner of holistic medicine,
for example on the American Holistic Medical Association
website.

These people are real specialists, usually treating complex
diseases, and they often don't take insurance. They rarely act
as primary care physicians because they are in such demand.
They will be too busy to respond if your child has a fever.

You are not asking the doctor to be the *expert* in natural
remedies – you just want a doctor who will *support* you in
your efforts.

A simple way to find someone like that is to ask at your local
independent health food store – the folks there are likely to
know who's in town.

Or ask a holistic professional who they refer to –
ask a trusted acupuncturist, chiropractor, homeopath,
naturopath, massage therapist or other professional if their
clients have a favorite physician.

Or ask the members of your local Holistic Moms group (see
page 119). HolisticMoms.org is a great way for like-minded
parents to share information like this.

# Find a Professional Homeopath

This book is meant to support you in treating *acute* conditions – that means things that just started within the past few days and are likely to go away on their own anyway within the next few weeks.

Homeopathy also works wonderfully for *chronic* conditions, ones that have been going on for a long time and will not resolve on their own. You'll need professional help for that.

First, let's be clear about what you want: "homeopathy" is often misused to mean "natural healing" in general. It's not – it's the little sugar pills that have been highly energized so they convey information to your body's healing energy.

A professional homeopath is someone who uses homeopathy as their only, or their primary, modality, not someone who does it as a little sideline to another practice like acupuncture or chiropractic.

A professional homeopath may or may not have a license in another health care modality (except in a couple of states, where they are required to be MDs).

There are advantages either way. A homeopath without a medical license *may* have more training in homeopathy, or more of a focus on homeopathy, than a medical professional (not necessarily, though). A medically-licensed homeopath could be better equipped to handle someone with a serious health problem on a lot of medications.

Here's what I feel is important. The homeopath must be well-trained, with lots of experience, a good track record for getting good results, and with a good bedside manner. She or he will need to ask you some really personal questions, and you need to feel comfortable answering them.

You'll be lucky if you can find this combination all in the same person. I think the best place to start is word of mouth: ask at your local health food store, and ask other practitioners like your chiropractor, acupuncturist or massage therapist.

One thing to look for – the credential CCH, which stands for Certified Classical Homeopath. This means the person is nationally certified after 1000 hours of training.

There are good homeopaths who do not have this credential, because they have been in practice so long they already had a well-established practice when the credential was created 20 years ago.

Or it could be because their practice is so busy they don't feel the need for the credential. This is especially true of MD homeopaths (ones that are licensed medical doctors as well as homeopaths). They are rare and you are lucky if you can find one!

You can find CCH-certified homeopaths at www.homeopathicdirectory.org.

There are only about 500 of us in the United States, so you may need to use my fallback option for finding a homeopath: word of mouth.

# How Do the Remedies Work?

People always ask me: how can homeopathy work if there's nothing in it?

There IS "something in it": information! Think of a remedy as a tiny computer chip. You could store a whole book on a computer chip, right?

A homeopathic remedy is a way of storing and transmitting information to your body's healing energy (Vital Force). It teaches the Vital Force a better way to deal with something that has made it go out of kilter or off balance. Then the Vital Force can let go of the symptoms it has created to restore the balance – and you feel better, naturally.

Think of the homeopath as a piano tuner and the conventional doctor as a carpenter. Most of the time, a piano can be tuned without needing any sawing or hammering. Maybe once in a while the piano has been damaged so that it needs to be repaired by the carpenter before being retuned.

In the same way, many health conditions can be addressed with the "re-tuning" of a homeopathic remedy. Sometimes – like if you've been in a car accident or if you've broken a bone – there's no substitute for surgery (the "carpenter").

But why not start with the simplest, safest and least invasive method first? Why not try the simple "re-tuning" of a homeopathic remedy before trying something more drastic?

We could save so much money in our health care system this way. But much more importantly, people would be healthier overall – because this kind of "re-tuning" creates *positive* side effects for the whole person.

## How can a remedy store information?

Snowflakes are all chemically identical: all are made out of water, $H_2O$. Yet their patterns are all different.

In the same way, the water of different homeopathic remedies is chemically identical, but the pattern of the water molecules is *different* in a way that stores information. Cutting-edge research in physics is documenting this effect of coherent or structured water.

Computers store huge amounts of information with a simple on-off (1 for on and 0 for off) method. Remedies are able to store huge amounts of information by changes in the orientation and bonding of simple water molecules.

The starting substance from which the remedy is made creates a pattern in the water molecules which is consistent for each remedy substance, and different from the pattern made by other remedy substances.

What happens once this information is transmitted to your body is still unknown. But then again, the mechanism of action of many of our common drugs is also unknown.


## How come I've never heard of homeopathy?

Homeopathy is the people's medicine. It's your medicine. The remedies are not patentable; they are in the public domain. A tube of a homeopathic remedy that costs $7.95 in a health food store can last you for years.

As a result, there are no extra funds generated to publicize homeopathy. Most people find out about it through word of mouth from satisfied users. Please tell your friends!

# What to Say to a Skeptic

I see a lot of contradictory arguments against homeopathy – that there's nothing in it, and that it's dangerous!

And a lot of critics say it's "unproven", which is not true – there is extensive research supporting it – but in any case, remember that "unproven" does not mean "proven not to work." It means "not tested yet", due to lack of funds.

It's also said to work by the placebo effect, but that cannot be true because it works on infants, animals, even on plants. Anyone who has given a remedy to a baby screaming with teething pain, and watched the child stop crying instantaneously, knows that it cannot possibly be the placebo effect.

Nor can the effect be based on a positive interaction with a professional homeopath, as some claim. (This is my father the doctor's theory! "You're a nice person and people like talking to you. That's why they feel better.") No matter how supportive the experience, no matter how much the client enjoys feeling truly heard, the recommended remedy will not work if it is not a good match for the client.

The best proof of homeopathy's effectiveness is personal experience. Try the remedies in this book. Sometimes homeopathy does not work well for a particular person, but if you keep trying it on several people, you *will* see it work.

There is plenty of research, though, most of it conducted overseas. Dana Ullman has done such an incredible job of keeping track of this research and describing it, that I'll simply refer you to his website, **www.homeopathic.com.**

If you would like to read a book about the research, it is well summarized in Dr. Bill Gray's *Homeopathy: Science or Myth* and in Dr. Amy Lansky's *Impossible Cure.*

For a thorough review of two centuries of research, please see Michael Emmans Dean's *The Trials of Homeopathy.* And for more about the science behind its mechanism of action, please see Bellavite and Signorini's *The Emerging Science of Homeopathy: Complexity, Biodynamics, and Nanopharmacology.*

## How come my doctor says it's unproven?

Chances are your doctor is not familiar with the research on homeopathy, which is not at all her/his fault, since most of the research has been done overseas and is not taught in American medical schools.

Homeopathic pharmacies cannot afford to fund research the way American drug companies do. The US government has funded a few studies which have demonstrated the effectiveness of homeopathy and have been published in peer-reviewed journals (for example, on homeopathy for childhood diarrhea and for mild traumatic brain injury).

To reassure your doctor, try telling her or him that homeopathy is an accepted part of the national health care system in many countries around the world and that the FDA treats it as a system of medicine, quite different from vitamins and herbs.

## Why is Wikipedia so negative about homeopathy?

The editorial board at Wikipedia (which is not as neutral as they would like us to believe) has recently been suppressing attempts by homeopaths to post accurate information. Please see www.homeopathic.com for more about this.

# Diving Deeper - Reference Books

Ready for more than what this book covers? Just plunge in!

The **Mastering Natural Remedies** series of DVDs, featuring internationally distinguished author and lecturer Miranda Castro. Filmed when Miranda was teaching in Boston, it includes her answers to practical questions from participants just like you. Miranda's seminars are vivid, entertaining, and full of stories that help you remember the remedies and how to use them. Available from www.GreenHealing.org.

**Homeopathy 101** covers basic first aid, accidents, injuries, preparing for surgery – much more detail, more conditions and more remedies than in this book.

**StressBusters** covers emotional traumas and remedies for all kinds of fears and anxieties, plus it explains our understanding of causation – the powerful paradigm of the Never Well Since.

**12 Gentle Souls, the Cell Salts** covers these universally useful, very low potency (really safe) remedies.
(this one only from www.MirandaCastro.com)


Other Healer In Every Home books:

**A Healer In Every Home – For Animals**

**A Healer In Every Home – Professional Version**

We'd like to notify you when these books become available. Please email us at books@greenhealing.org and we'll let you know as soon as they're ready.

**More reference books:**

Here are suggestions, available from Homeopathic
Educational Services, **www.homeopathic.com.** This is
the best source because they have so many resources and
so much free information about homeopathy.

For your next book, I would get **Everybody's Guide to
Homeopathic Medicines** by Cummngs and Ullman. It
covers many more conditions than we cover here, and gives
more remedy options for the conditions in this book.
I like it because for each condition it has a section called
"Beyond Home Care." This tells you the warning signs that
you should call your doctor, head for the hospital, or even
call 911.

If you have kids, please also get Dana Ullman's
**Homeopathic Medicines for Children and Infants.**
It has lots more information about the conditions and
the remedies most likely to be needed when treating kids.

Another favorite – Dennis Chernin's **Complete
Homeopathic Resource for Common Illnesses.**
Thorough and clear, written by a homeopathic MD.

When you feel ready for the "advanced course", get
Miranda Castro's **Complete Handbook of Homeopathy.**
You can get it free from her website, www.MirandaCastro.com,
when you get the Miranda Castro Kit, which has all the
remedies recommended in her book.

If you are pregnant or have a newborn, the best "advanced
course" book is Miranda Castro's **Homeopathy for
Pregnancy, Birth and Your Baby's First Year.**

# Books to Enjoy Reading

While the books recommended in the previous section were reference books to dip into as needed, these books are fun to keep on your nightstand or even take to the beach.

**Impossible Cure** by Dr. Amy Lansky
A NASA computer scientist, Amy turned to homeopathy when her son was diagnosed with autism.

Of course, conventional medicine has no treatment for autism, let alone holding out hope of a cure – but her son was completely cured with homeopathy.

Amy was so impressed that she left NASA and trained to become a professional homeopath herself. As a scientist, she was especially interested in the research behind homeopathy – both how it works (its "mechanism of action") and how it fares in research trials with particular diseases.

In this book, she alternates the story of her son's cure with clear and easy to understand descriptions of the research on homeopathy.

This is my favorite introductory book to explain how homeopathy works.

**Nature and Human Personality** by Catherine Coulter.
The major homeopathic remedies are not only powerful curative agents, they also have personality types associated with them – like the whiny, clingy, cuddly Pulsatilla, the tantruming and impossible-to-please Chamomilla, or the irritable, ambitious and competitive Nux vomica.

This book is just plain fun to read. You will recognize your family members, your friends and coworkers in its pages.

The fact that these "remedy pictures" are so true to life helps underscore the natural laws that homeopathy follows.

**The Homeopathic Revolution** by Dana Ullman. This describes all the famous people in the past 200 years who used homeopathy – even whose lives were saved by homeopathy (Darwin for example!).
Whether you admire Popes or pop stars, you'll find some of your heroes here.
And if you have a skeptic in the house, telling him that his favorite soccer star uses homeopathy might help turn him around!

**The A Cappella Singer Who Lost Her Voice and Other Stories from Natural Medicine** by Dr. Amy Rothenberg. In the style of the Oliver Sacks books, this book teaches through stories.
In the process of telling these enjoyable stories – most of which are from the field of homeopathy – Dr. Rothenberg introduces you to a new way of thinking about the body and healing, plus she shares lots of practical tips and resources.

# Books About Specific Topics

**First Aid**
If you expect to find yourself in emergency situations a lot, you should get *Help! and Homeopathy: What to Do In an Emergency Until 911 Arrives* by Eileen Naumann, a homeopath who works as an EMT. It has lots of practical advice for dealing with emergencies in addition to remedy recommendations.

Note: Some of the following books give information about treating **chronic (longterm) conditions.** Please do not treat yourself or others for these conditions – go to a professional homeopath instead (see page 108). Instead, please take this information as inspiring examples of what homeopathy can do.

**Emotional First Aid/Treating Emotional Trauma**
*A Homeopathic Guide to Stress* by Miranda Castro
*Prozac-Free* by Robert Ullman and Judyth Reichenberg-Ullman
*Emotional Healing with Homeopathy* by Peter Chappell
*Homeopathy for the Soul* by Cassandra Lorius

**Children's Conditions**
*Ritalin-Free Kids* and *Rage-Free Kids* by Robert Ullman and Judyth Reichenberg-Ullman

**Women's Issues**
*Whole Woman Homeopathy* by Judyth Reichenberg-Ullman
*Beauty in Bloom* by Eileen Naumann (about menopause)

**Science and Research on Homeopathy**
*Homeopathy: Science or Myth?* by Bill Gray
*Homeopathic Family Medicine* by Dana Ullman (this ebook includes extensive scientific references)

# Websites to Explore

These are just a few of my favorites. Tell us yours and we may include them in the next edition!

**www.homeopathic.org** has lots of great information about homeopathy; join the National Center for Homeopathy via this site and you'll get a beautiful bimonthly journal.

**www.NourishMD.com** is a website run by a pediatrician and a holistic nutritionist. These terrific women are both moms and their website focuses on healthy food and supplements and how to get kids to eat or take them!

**www.HolisticMoms.org** is both an online community and in some locales, a meet-up group. For years I've heard moms in my practice say, "I'm the only mother I know who is trying to keep her kids off sugar and off the computer, feed them healthy food, get them outside to play . . ." and I've wished I could get these moms together, but they lived too far apart.
Now Holistic Moms is creating this kind of community. It's a great way to share information, true – but more importantly, it creates emotional support for all of you who feel like you're swimming upstream in this heavily commercialized culture.

**www..hookedonnature.org, www.childrenandnature. org** about encouraging kids to go out in nature, invoking Richard Louv's *Last Child in the Woods.*

**www.DrMercola.com, www.NaturalNews.com** Lots of important information about natural alternatives to drugs. Dr. Mercola and Mike Adams (on NaturalNews) have excellent information; just be cautious about the ads, and the "Citizen Journalist" stories on NaturalNews.com.

# Support Your Body's Healing Energy

Homeopathy works with the body's own natural healing energy (called the Vital Force in homeopathy and *chi* in Traditional Chinese Medicine). The more of this healing energy you have, the more effectively the remedy can work. If your Vital Force is weak, here are some ways you can strengthen it.

My personal favorite and something I recommend to everyone – the **Donna Eden 5-Minute Daily Energy Routine.** It really does take just 5 minutes! (well, maybe 10 because you'll enjoy it so much you'll want to linger over it). You can see my friend Karen Semmelman demonstrate it on the GreenHealingTV channel on YouTube! Look for the Energy episode.

**Other energy-based exercises** such as yoga, Tai Chi, Qi Gong, aikido, and the Tibetan Five Rites can strengthen your healing energy. Personally I find Tai Chi hard to follow, but I find Qi Gong easy and just as effective.

The Tibetan Five Rites, also easy, are described in *The Fountain of Youth*, available in health food stores, or search YouTube for demonstration videos. Many people have found that they restore youthfulness.

**Diet:** Eat fresh, pure foods as much as possible. Try to feel how much life-energy a food has before deciding whether to eat it. Raw fruits and vegetables are ideal; make juices of them if they are hard to digest whole.

You know what's made the biggest difference for me?

Remember I've been a vegetarian, natural/organic foods eater for 40 years, and my diet still needed improving.

I got a Vita-Mix and followed the "green smoothie" recipes demonstrated by Victoria Boutenko on YouTube. Try them – they're delicious and kids really like them!

Avoid foods with lots of sugar and white flour, fat, and chemicals, i.e. all junk and processed foods.

However, it is also important to enjoy what you eat so you may need to make this transition gradually. Try to explore new foods until you find things you really like which are also healthy.

**Deep breathing** of fresh pure air will bring *prana* or life-energy into your system.

Avoid conventional fluorescent lights; use **natural spectrum lights**.

**Pure water:** Use a really good water filter, since tap water in many cities has been found to contain chemicals including pharmaceuticals.

**Flowers and nature:** Go out in nature, walk barefoot in the grass (if safe/practical), feel the healing energy of the earth. Keep fresh flowers in your room. Tend a garden and feel the living, growing energy of the little shoots as they push up. Human beings need to stay connected with the energy of the earth. If you're a city-dweller, get an Earthing Mat from www.earthing.net. Mine has made a huge difference for me!

**Spiritual practices:** Your own prayer and meditation can help. You can ask your family, friends and congregation or spiritual community to pray for you. For example, if you are going through surgery, have it announced during services so that people can pray for you at that particular time.

I heard Dr. Larry Dossey on PBS describe a study he did on the power of prayer. Patients recovering from surgery in a hospital were divided into two groups – half of them were prayed for by people who didn't know them, the other half were not, and in all other ways the groups were similar. The patients didn't know if they were being prayed for or not.

Do you know, the patients who were prayed for got better faster, were discharged from the hospital sooner, had fewer complications and needed less pain medication?
Dr. Dossey said, "If a medication got results like this, it would immediately be adopted by every hospital in the country!"

**Meditation** can be very helpful – to bring you peace of mind and to help focus your healing energy on a remedy when you are giving it to someone, or taking it yourself.

My spiritual teacher, Sri Chinmoy, used to suggest praying for someone, then feeling that you are putting the power of your prayer into the remedy itself as you give it to them. This is an especially effective way to connect with your family members as you are treating them. It's also a great way to remember that ultimately we are not doing the healing – we are just the instruments of a higher power.

The heart-center meditation of Sri Chinmoy is a wonderful way to connect with your own higher power.
I teach **free classes in heart-center meditation** in the Boston area. See www.FreeMeditationBoston.org.

You can find free classes in other cities, taught by my friends in the Sri Chinmoy Centre, at
www.SriChinmoyCentre.org.

They are all offered as a community service and the teachers do not accept donations.

## About the Author

Begabati was born into a medical family: her father, a vascular surgeon, ran a vascular research lab where he tested the prototype model for the Doppler ultrasound device. Her mother was a research biochemist who researched stains for Dr. Papanicolau while he was developing the Pap smear. (Her mother's promising career came to an untimely end with the arrival of Begabati; her mother had a second career later in life as a nature-loving third grade teacher.)

Her parents were also early conservationists and Audubon enthusiasts. When Begabati was 8, they had landscapers create a wildflower garden for her in the back yard, complete with a map with the botanical names of all the plants. (To her delight, these same plants showed up later in her life as medicinal herbs and homeopathic remedies.)

Begabati entered Harvard in 1969 planning to become a doctor like her dad, but she developed a passionate commitment for natural healing as an undergraduate, and her life took a different turn. At a time when there was no professional training in natural medicine, she graduated from Harvard with a junior-year Phi Beta Kappa (putting her in the top 1% of her class) and opened a health food store.

Begabati ran her health food store until she was 40, interacting with thousands of customers and developing a treasure trove of knowledge about natural remedies – from her studies and, more importantly, from talking to customers about what worked for them and how they could tell.

Turning 40 and determined to pursue professional training in natural healing, she chose homeopathy as by far the most effective of the modalities in her health food store. She was impressed by both the speed of its action in acute cases and the depth of its reach in chronic cases. It could resolve trauma from the person's early childhood, and it could heal emotional problems in a way that vitamins and herbs could not.

Begabati co-founded the Renaissance Institute of Classical Homeopathy in 1996 with her mentor, the internationally-distinguished homeopath Dr. Luc De Schepper. She served as administrator of the school until 2001, while it was in Boston. She was Director of Teleosis School of Homeopathy, a professional training program, from 2003 to 2010.

In 2011 she turned her focus to educating and empowering a wider audience in basic home health care with natural remedies, by founding the GreenHealing Institute. She also practices classical homeopathy at the Lydian Center for Innovative Medicine in Cambridge, Mass.

A former professional editor and graphic designer, Begabati has edited a number of top reference books in homeopathy for well-known American and European authors. She was the co-author with Dr. June Riedlinger of the Homeopathy chapter in the American Pharmacists Association's *Handbook of Non-Prescription Drugs.*

Mostly, though, she likes to teach and to share what she knows. She lectures on homeopathy at Massachusetts College of Pharmacy and Health Sciences and at Lesley University. You can see her passion for natural healing in action in her community-access TV show, *A Healer In Every Home,* on the GreenHealingTV channel on YouTube.

Begabati loves being an aunt. She especially loves it when her four-year-old niece Sally says, "I need my Begabati medicine!"

# Index of Conditions

abandoned, feeling, 91
abdominal surgery 18
allergic reactions, 77
anesthesia, recovery from 22
anxiety, 9, 35, 52, 62
    before the dentist, exams,
      or vet (for pets) 62
appendicitis, 84

back pain, 71, 83
bee stings, 78
bladder infections, 10, 71. 78
black eyes, 16
bleeding, 28
breast injuries, 18
broken bones, 73, 84
bruises, 11

canker sores, 83
chicken pox, 72, 78, 83
childbirth, 16, 18
chills, 57
cold sores, 83
cold wind, 9
colds, 10, 45–46, 53–54, 71
colic, 40
coughs, 29–30, 40–53, 71, 84
concussion, 16
conjunctivitis, 10, 53, 78, 91
constipation, 70, 84
cramps, 40, 70
crisis, 40
croup, 10
cuts, 21, 28

dental extractions, 16, 22
diarrhea, 53, 62, 70, 91
digestive problems, 70
dizziness, 62

ear infections, 10, 91
electrical shocks, 29
episiotomy, 32
eye with foreign
    object in it, 10
emergency, 5–7
emotional upsets, 36–37
exhaustion, 52

fever, 10, 57, 62, 78, 91
fever blisters, 83
food poisoning, 67
flu, 10, 15, 53, 57–59, 62,
    71, 83, 91
fractures, 76, 84
fright, 9
fungus under the nails, 80

gums, bleeding 29

hair, brittle, 81
hangovers, 70
hay fever, 53, 62, 71
headaches, 53, 84
hearing bad news, 36, 62
heartburn, 70
hemorrhoids, 29, 70
herpes, 78
high altitudes, 76

hives, 77
hoarseness, 29, 83
humiliation, 36

impetigo, 83
infection prevention, 21
insomnia, 40, 53, 62
insect bites, 78, 80

jet lag, 15, 76
joint pain, 83–85

kidney stones, 71

laryngitis, 10
lightning, 29
lump in the throat, 40

mammograms, 18
mastitis, 84
menstrual bleeding, 28
menstrual cramps, 71, 78
middle of night, 9
mouth sores 53
mucus 45–46
muscle cramps, 40, 71

nails, brittle, 81
nausea, 40, 53, 67–69
nerve pain, 33–34
nerve–rich areas, 33–34
nerves, frazzled 34
nosebleeds, 16, 28

panic, 6
pain, 21–22
phantom limb pain, 33
poison ivy or oak, 83
postpartum hemorrhage, 28

potty training, 89, 91–92
psychosomatic symptoms, 40
puncture wounds, 33
rashes, 78
rectal spasms, 40

scarring, 21, 26
sciatica, 33–34
scrapes, 21
shingles, 53, 83
sore throat, 10, 53, 72, 83
spasms, 40
spine injuries, 32–33
splinters, 81
sports injuries, 11
sprains, 82–84
strains, 82–84
stage fright, 62
stings, 71
stomach cramps, 70
stomachache, 91
surgery, 22–27

teething, 89–91
toilet training, 89, 91, 93
tonsillitis, 78
tooth extraction, 22
tooth pain, 32
trauma, 7, 11, 36
travelers' diarrhea, 53

vertigo, 62
vomiting, 40, 53, 67–79

water retention, 78
whiplash, 83
wound healing, 21

# Index of Remedies and Supplements

Aconite 5–7, 9–10
Allium cepa, 45, 88
Apis, 66–67
Arnica, 11–12, 14–15, 17, 20, 51, 65
Arsenicum, 40, 46–47, 51, 65, 75

Bellis perennis, 17
Bryonia, 71, 73

Calc fluor, 13
Calc phos, 80
Calendula, 19–20, 65
Calms Forte 34–35
Carbo veg, 76
Chamomilla, 89–90
China (Cinchona) 104
Cocculus, 104

Elderberry, 51
Emergen–C, 51

Ferrum phos, 60

Gelsemium, 36–39, 57, 62

Hepar sulph, 45
Hypericum, 33–34
Hyland's Teething Tablets, 95

Ignatia, 37–42
Influenzinum, 59

Joint Cream, 85–86

Kali bic, 45. 47
Kali phos, 34

Mag phos, 75

Nerve Tonic, 341
No Jet Lag, 104

Nux vomica, 58, 67–69, 72

Oscillococcinum, 59

Phosphorus, 22, 28–29, 76
Pulsatilla, 67, 89–94

Rescue Remedy 7, 43–44
Rhus tox, 82–83
Rutin, 14

Seven Cream, 80
Silica 81
Sulphur, 8
Symphytum, 73

Traumeel, 14–15